Now or Never?

Having a Baby Later in Life

by

Yvonne Bostock and Maggie Jones

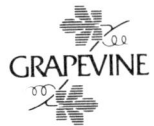

GRAPEVINE

First published 1987

British Library Cataloguing in Publication Data

Bostock, Yvonne
  Now or never? : having a baby later in life.
  1. Pregnancy in middle age   2. Childbirth in middle age
  I. Title   II. Jones, Maggie
  618.2′00240431   RG556.6

ISBN 0-7225-1355-0

*Grapevine is part of the Thorsons Publishing Group,
Wellingborough, Northamptonshire, NN8 2RQ, England*

Printed in Great Britain by
Hazell, Watson and Viney Limited,
Member of BPCC plc, Aylesbury, Buckinghamshire

10 9 8 7 6 5 4 3 2

Contents

Introduction: The older mother   9

Chapter One: Having a baby – planned and unplanned   13
*first reactions *attitudes *advantages

Chapter Two: Pregnancy and looking after yourself   26
*stopping contraception *avoiding drugs in pregnancy
*diet during pregnancy *preconceptual care *keeping fit in
pregnancy *antenatal care *finding out you are pregnant
*routine antenatal tests *twin pregnancies *emotional
changes in pregnancy *sex in pregnancy

Chapter Three: Still not pregnant   43
*am I fertile? *how to get pregnant *time to get help
*getting medical help *the causes of infertility *infertility
tests *treatments for infertility in women *treatments for
infertility in men *problems with infertility investigations
*miscarriage

Chapter Four: Screening for abnormalities   65
*how the baby develops *how things go wrong *Down's
Syndrome *neural tube defects *cleft lip and palate
*abnormalities of the digestive tract *detecting abnormalities
*if something goes wrong

Chapter Five: Having the baby   83
*how labour begins *special risks for the older mother
*pain relief in labour *difficult labours *medical
intervention *the premature delivery *care of the premature
baby *stillbirth *bonding with your baby *breast feeding
*the post-natal check

Chapter Six: Afterwards   110
                   *emotional and physical reactions   *support   *older children
                   *going back to work   *weaning to go back to work   *planning
                   to be a working mother   *maternity leave and pay   *being a
                   full time mother   *Adapting, the new roles and sharing the
                   responsibility

Further reading   135
Useful addresses   137
Index   141

For
Joanna, Camilla and Jay
&
Edward and Toby

Having a baby at any age is one of the most exciting times in any woman's life; and for a couple – young or maybe not so young – starting or adding to their family, the prospect is one of quite dramatic changes in their life and new responsibilities.

More women than ever before are having babies in 'later life' or, more precisely, over the age of 30. This trend has increased over the last 10 years, and figures also show that women have been having their babies later and later. The number of first babies born to women who have been married for between 10 and 14 years has doubled during that time, and there has been a marked increase in the number of births to unmarried professional women in their thirties*

Yet having a baby is one of the most down-to-earth, everyday, run-of-the-mill occurrences which for so long has been largely taken for granted. Until very recently it was generally assumed that most women would marry at a young age and that children would quickly follow – if, indeed, a baby was not already on the way. A childless couple would have been

*New Society 1/11/1985.

looked on with sympathy but little help would have been offered to assess the reason why the woman had failed to conceive. Most would never have thought to seek medical help and a childless couple would simply have accepted their distress and grief as the 'luck of the draw'. But a post-war generation of women has lived through social and economic changes which have greatly affected their lives in general and their ability to choose when they would start families. Having a choice over whether and when to have children has profoundly changed people's attitudes to marriage, child rearing and family life.

The 1950s and '60s in this country were a time of economic growth, jobs for all and more career opportunities for women. The contraceptive pill was a major breakthrough in allowing many women to control their fertility. But as the '60s gave way to the '70s, inflation, the rising cost of living and the rising costs of property and mortgages brought a new economic dimension to marriage itself. More young couples felt that two incomes rather than one were needed to sustain a reasonable standard of living.

Increasingly, young couples chose to postpone starting a family for a few years. More and more working women recognized that their contribution was of equal value to that of their male counterparts and their commitment to careers became less easy to surrender. Many would say that, as a society, we came to value work inside the home less and less. Being 'a housewife' was to be stripped of status and, some have argued, identity as well. Women who once would have found fulfilment in the home and in the role of wife and mother, went in search of identities, satisfaction and self-fulfilment.

During the same period there have been dramatic changes in society's view of marriage itself. Only a generation ago it was thought of as almost sacrosanct. Today, one in three marriages ends in divorce, although marriage as an institution remains popular – statistics show that the majority of people who divorce will remarry, most of these marriages constituting step-families. So while patterns of family life may have changed, the view of normal family life still centres around marriage. Whether or not there are children from previous marriages, a newly married couple often want a child of their own to cement their relationship.

But not everyone marries and there are a small but growing number of single older women who are not in a steady relationship, either through varied circumstances or by preference, and who are just as keen to have a baby and bring it up with or without the involvement of the father.

All this has meant that more and more women who put off having children in their twenties are opting for motherhood, or are getting pregnant again in their mid to late thirties and more women are having second families in their late thirties or even early forties. Yet from a medical point of view, much of the evidence relating to the best age for a woman to have a baby still points to the early to mid twenties as being the 'prime time'. Evidence about the incidence of handicap, such as Down's Syndrome and other genetic disorders, has been presented very simply and somewhat negatively – suggesting that every woman over the age of 35 who has a baby is at risk. No one would want to dismiss these risks, but nor would they want to cause unnecessary worry. True, the risk does increase with age, but set against this the chances are that a woman will have a perfectly healthy baby at any age.

The fact is that there are very many women getting pregnant in their thirties and forties for all sorts of reasons. Most are aware that in delaying pregnancy certain risks are involved. But they also consider these risks to be worth taking. For these women the social and emotional considerations are no less important than the purely medical ones. Some have problems with their pregnancies, others have none; but most have perfectly normal, healthy babies.

Women often also feel pressurized by society, family and friends to have a baby before they are 'too old' – 'too old' often meaning over 30 and certainly over 35. However, as so much evidence shows, having a baby later on is not as risky as is often thought. Added to this, very many older couples find that there are considerable benefits in delaying having children. Their own maturity and confidence often gives them great satisfaction and pleasure in doing a job which they would have been less well prepared for earlier in their lives.

In the course of writing this book we talked to many women who had had a baby when in their thirties or forties. All their situations were different. Some were apprehensive because of their age and what they knew about being an 'elderly primipara' and suffered agonies awaiting the outcome of tests. Several conceived and finally produced their babies after long and distressing periods of infertility investigations. Others had straightforward normal pregnancies with no such problems or apprehensions. Not all the pregnancies were planned. But these women had one thing in common – their babies were all wanted babies.

Table 1: Live births, age of mother   England and Wales

Year	All ages	Under 20	20-24	25-29	30-34	35-39	40-44	45 and over
	All live births							
1974	639,885	68,725	208,084	235,593	89,132	30,308	7,496	548
1975	603,445	63,507	190,198	225,990	88,379	28,147	6,653	571
1976	584,270	57,943	182,210	220,712	90,791	26,117	5,999	498
1977	569,259	54,477	174,544	207,916	100,807	25,527	5,534	454
1978	596,418	55,984	182,580	210,598	113,077	27,937	5,719	523
1979	638,028	59,143	193,209	222,102	125,664	31,394	5,978	538
1980	656,234	60,754	201,541	223,438	129,908	33,893	6,075	625
1981	634,492	56,570	194,500	215,760	126,590	34,210	6,170	690
1982	625,931	55,435	192,322	211,905	120,758	38,992	5,886	633
1983	629,134	54,059	191,852	214,078	120,996	41,277	6,210	662
1984	636,818	54,508	191,455	218,031	122,774	42,921	6,576	553
1985	656,417	56,929	193,958	227,486	126,185	44,393	6,882	584
1986	661,018	57,406	192,064	229,035	129,487	45,465	7,033	528

NB. 1981 births for age groups are based on a 10 per cent sample.
Source: OPCS.

CHAPTER ONE

Having a Baby — planned and unplanned

For many couples, having a baby when the woman is over the age of 30 is a conscious choice and part of a deliberate plan to put off having a family until other things have been achieved or accomplished. For some, tied to jobs or other commitments, it is not so much a choice as the inevitable way in which things happen in their lives. Where one or both partners is marrying for the second time, couples often want a child of their own to cement the relationship. Women with children almost grown find that the temptation to add to their families while they still can becomes a pressing need in their late thirties or early forties. Other women, who consider themselves long past late-night feeds, nappies and the demands of a small baby – and possibly adjusting to the slower, quieter and more dignified pace of a middle-aged life style – suddenly, unexpectedly and unintentionally find themselves pregnant.

Yet, despite the fact that having a baby later in life is increasingly commonplace, figures themselves tell us nothing about how women feel about postponing pregnancy, how they feel about being an 'older mother' and just how easy the decision to have a baby, or to go ahead with a pregnancy, may or may not be.

Some couples are lucky in that they do have the planned-for baby later, as hoped and intended. In Jean's case the choice was a very deliberate one on the part of her and her husband. He owned a plot of land on a beautiful site in a lovely setting but within easy reach of the centre of the city in which they both worked. They decided to build a house on the land and spent several years working weekends and evenings on the building project. It was a massive undertaking; with no capital, every penny that Jean earned went into buying building materials. Bill's salary kept them – a case of 'build as you earn'. Once they had made up their minds that this was the only way they could hope to have a home of their own without a massive mortgage round their neck. Jean and Bill kept to their agreement.

Building their own house was sufficient reason for this couple to postpone parenthood. Yet they admit that it wasn't just a matter of building a house. Both needed time to get to know each other and make sure that they were right for each other. Jean says that she was not ready to have a family at 26 and she was quite happy to put it off for a while. However, the decision was not entirely free from worry and some apprehension did build up over time:

> It did worry me for a year or two before, you know – 'What happens if we run into problems?' I could easily have been forty before I had my first child. It was always at the back of our minds and obviously, as the years went by, we were getting too old to adopt so we could have had quite a problem on our hands.

It would be easy to say that Jean had no reason to worry, since, when they did decide to go ahead and have a baby, it did not take very long for Jean to conceive. There was, of course, no way she could know that and the concern was something she had to live with – all part of the 'calculated risk'.

The apprehension for women trying to have a first baby over 30 stems from the fear of the unknown. As one woman put it: 'If you haven't put yourself to the test yet, you don't know that everything is OK.'

The decision to work for a few years after marriage to get established and set up home is one which many newly married women make. For others it is less of a choice and more an economic necessity. Liz worked full time for four years before she had her first baby at 31:

> 'We were married in 1973 when prices were high – it was an expensive time and prices of houses were going up. Fortunately, we had no problems when we did decide to start a family – I got pregnant straight away.'

Like many others, both these women had their 'planned' babies at a time in their lives when they wanted them. It is reassuring to think that life can be so controlled and organized, but in practice there are very many women who have to wait some considerable time before they get pregnant – and this can be harrowing as months pass by and the sense of time 'running out' begins to make itself felt. Diminishing fertility may be a problem for women approaching their forties and it requires no small commitment and dedication for a couple to go through the process of infertility testing and treatments.

Repeated miscarriages can also cause a great deal of distress for a small minority of women. This was Heather's problem. After three miscarriages in her mid-thirties, she was told she should wait some time before trying again:

> I was beginning to think it was all too much trouble and I was upset and I didn't really want another baby but I didn't want to go back on the pill. So we agreed to use sheaths and I said, 'Right, it's your responsibility.' He wasn't very good at it and I was pregnant with Margaret! She was an accident after three miscarriages!

A baby can be wanted in later life for reasons which could never have been foreseen earlier in life or 'planned' for. Second marriages, as a result of divorce or bereavement, can dramatically change the best-laid plans. Sarah was married for a second time after being widowed and left with two teenage children from her first marriage. Sarah's second husband had no children of his own and they both very much wanted a child. At 36 the planned-for baby was conceived. But, while she was delighted to be pregnant, Sarah was nervous about the birth. She had been told, after two very difficult pregnancies in her twenties, that she would always have to have a forceps delivery: 'But I felt great – normal morning sickness, normal delivery... and that after having been told that I would always have to have forceps.'

Many babies born to older mothers are definitely not planned, but what may begin as an error often turns out to be what one couple described as 'the best mistake we ever made'. Two years after having James, Sarah discovered she was pregnant again – this time by accident:

After James was born I had a coil fitted, which was great and very successful until last year when I started having pains and feeling very unwell... I was finally referred to the hospital who thought it might be a tubal pregnancy or chronic infection due to the coil. So I had the coil removed and they told me that, 'with your age and diminishing fertility, and until you've made up your mind about sterilization, sheaths should be all right!' This baby is the result of diminishing fertility!

But a couple making a go of marriage for a second time don't always want children. Some will be quite sure about this, while others may not have given it much thought, and only when a pregnancy occurs do they face up to the situation and consider what they really do want.

For Kathy, getting pregnant at the age of 38 was not what she had planned. She had remarried in her mid-thirties, having had a daughter at the age of 21. Her determination not to get pregnant meant that she had carried on taking the pill for some years. However, Kathy's doctor was concerned that, as a heavy smoker, she should think seriously about coming off the pill or giving up smoking. At the time there was no way that she would even think about giving up her cigarettes. So Kathy came off the pill and, as she puts it:

We struggled along with contraception, but it wasn't very satisfactory. We just took a risk. There was so much talk about infertility and how couples were trying for families and I think the older you get the less fertile you are. I had never taken risks and I think I felt, 'Well, it could never possibly happen this once,'... and it did and that rocked me to my foundations as well. I couldn't believe that it had happened to me.

Clearly, very many pregnancies begin as so-called 'accidents', or the result of failed contraception or in other situations where pregnancy is thought to be unlikely. Taking a chance with contraception can be just as risky for a woman of 38 as for an eighteen-year-old.

At the age of 42, Lynn found herself in a similar situation. She decided to come off the pill, having been on it for a long time. Her two daughters by her first marriage were aged fourteen and fifteen at the time. Her second husband was a few years younger than Lynn and he had made the decision that he did not want children of his own. Lynn came off the pill, quite sure that, in her own words, 'nothing could happen to me now.' Initially her weight gain was a minor concern. She had always had a tendency to gain weight rapidly. When it became a real problem she considered dieting, but the thought also occurred to her that she might be pregnant. She got in touch with her GP who confirmed her suspicions. It was quite a shock to discover that she was in fact 24 weeks pregnant.

Couples who get together while still very young may be no clearer ten years later about when to start a family, which is how Alison describes her situation. They were married while still in their twenties. Both Alison and her husband were successful musicians and although Alison says she desperately wanted children at that time, it was too unrealistic. Five years later she was having such a good time in her career, as she says, that:

> ... the idea would have been too constricting. But as I approached 40 I realized that we had better have children soon. We tried half-heartedly but I didn't conceive until I was 38 ... we weren't really planning it. It was a mixture of never being sure at the same time that we wanted children until it became necessary to have them because I was getting on. I think I was scared of the responsibility.

For the woman in her mid-thirties or more who is unmarried or whose partner does not want children, the choice of having a baby usually does not exist. There are women, however, who do decide to 'go it alone' and have a baby, either with the consent of their steady partner although he does not want to take on a paternal role, or through a casual sexual contact or even Artificial Insemination by Donor (AID).

> I'm now 40 and my chances of having a child are fading fast. For the past three years I've had a married lover with teenage children and he says he doesn't want to leave his wife or have more children. I've agonised over it a thousand times. As I see it, he has everything his way and I have nothing mine. I've told him I would never have an abortion; if I got pregnant by accident he would have to accept the fact of the baby's existence even if he decided to have nothing to do with it, which I wouldn't mind. Is it so very wrong?

Many women in such a position are worried about the effect that being without a father would have on the child. Having a child on its own is seen by most to be very selfish and manipulative. Yet, as one woman puts it, 'Men want a sexual relationship with no risk of having a child, but that is a very recent possibility. I think it is a man's view to think that its wrong for a woman to have a baby alone if she wants to and can take good care of it.'

Others find deep-seated beliefs about parenting are hard to change:

I thought about it, but at the end of the day I just knew in my heart that the best way to want a child is for that child's own sake. The best thing you can do for any child is to make sure it has the love of both parents. I want a child as much as any woman and while it looks like there might be two options – for me there's only one choice.

First reactions

Planned, unplanned or surprise pregnancy – whatever the circumstances, the popular notion is that when a woman discovers she is pregnant, (unless unmarried) she is immediately filled with a sense of maternal pleasure and happiness. Certainly no words can describe the sheer elation when a pregnancy is finally confirmed and the longed-for baby is on its way – and this is particularly so if a couple have tried for years for a pregnancy or have gone through the agonies of infertility problems. But not everyone feels joy and pleasure initially and women may have many different feelings and reactions – a confusion of what a child means to the woman herself, to the couple, to their situation and expectations. There may be some doubts and reservations, about reordering life around another person, bringing up the child and interrupting or giving up jobs and careers.

For the most part, these feelings change over time as the couple adapt, adjust and reappraise their situation. In some cases, as for Kathy, first reactions may mean coming to terms with an unwanted major upheaval in their lives. Only when they have worked through the disappointment and seen that they can reorder their lives, are they able to allow themselves to enjoy their pregnancy.

Kathy admits that at first she was not very happy and things could have worked out very badly for her as her husband had just accepted a job posting abroad:

I felt resentment initially. It wasn't what I wanted and we had all these plans. I was offered a termination. But Ron had no family of his own and when I sat down and thought about it, I couldn't do it . . . I couldn't abort it. If it had just been me I might have done it, but he was so pleased about it that I couldn't do it. It's turned out to be the best thing, really. I'm thrilled to bits. But I never would have planned it. It was a happy accident, really.

Ann, who had her first baby at the age of 38, confesses that, before she actually had children, she didn't think a great deal about how she would feel. She also adds that only after her first daughter did she realize how much she wanted a family: 'I don't know what would have happened if I hadn't; I suppose I would have blamed myself. To be honest, I wasn't really terribly keen on children as such, but having had her I wouldn't have missed it. I enjoyed her tremendously.'

Three miscarriages in rapid succession meant that when Heather got pregnant for a fourth time she was desperately anxious for the first few weeks. The previous miscarriages had created tensions for both her and her husband:

> I was beginning to get worried that I was beginning to get old and Peter wasn't that keen on having any more anyway. So we just left it at that. When I did get pregnant (by accident), the first few weeks were desperately anxious. Peter was annoyed – he was having enormous problems at work. He wanted to pack up his job and didn't feel that he could with a pregnant wife ... it was all a bit awful but he did get used to the idea.

For Heather it was a case of fourth time lucky – this time she did not miscarry.

Being pregnant 'by accident' can initially be more of an embarrassment than an occasion for celebrating, as Sarah pointed out:

> We were having a holiday without the children and I was feeling sick and dizzy. It was just before Sam's third birthday and I was feeling bloated. It all happened instantly – like turning on a switch.
>
> I went along with great embarrass-

ment to the clinic and there was a youngish doctor there. He was very good and very positive. I felt that when you get to my stage of life and you have three children you should have all this pretty well organized ... it was the failed contraception that I felt embarrassed about. I thought the doctor, who was so young, would be quietly sniggering behind his hand. But he was great! He said there would be very little difference between how I felt and how I coped having Sam and this one. I came away feeling very positive.

Initially, the doctor's reaction to Sarah who went along to see him with a bad case of 'failed contraception', was important in putting her at ease and dealing positively with her pregnancy. It perhaps also illustrates that a woman having a baby in her late thirties is not an oddity, and that attitudes generally are not necessarily what most women expect. But clearly other people's reactions can be quite important in influencing how a woman feels at first about being pregnant as an older mother.

Attitudes

When Jean, at 35, went along to see her doctor, he was delighted for her: 'He had been nagging at me for years and pushing – "You're not getting any younger!" He jokingly called me "an elderly prim". He obviously had no doubts about my health and was delighted that I had gone and done it!"

Jean went along to the maternity hospital for her first check-up and was pleasantly surprised that while she says she felt 'old', the doctors and nurses were unconcerned about her age. Her own attitude was that she 'didn't want to risk anything' and, because of her age and what she had read about the risks associated with pregnancy for older women, she was worried about the possibility of the baby being handicapped. For these reasons she had gone along to her first ante-natal appointment determined to have an amniocentesis:

I was determined to have it because I felt old and didn't want to risk anything. I felt the least I could do, having left it so long, was to be careful. They didn't offer it to me and I asked because I was so worried, but was told that they don't do it until 37, because you have to weigh up the dangers of it. At 35 the risk of amniocentesis triggering a miscarriage is greater than the risk of an abnormal baby, and it is possible that you would not conceive again. Well, this was a thing I had never thought of – it was an aspect I had not considered until then. They seemed so confident that eventually I agreed to give it a miss. But I was a little worried about it and I asked to see the consultant (up to then I had been seeing this very junior doctor). When I did see the consultant he said, 'There's absolutely nothing wrong with you. You're going to have the most super easy birth' – and he was absolutely right!

The fact that the consultant never made an issue about her age but put a lot of store by the fact that she was physically in good shape and was having a perfectly normal healthy pregnancy was very reassuring for Jean.

Obviously the responsibility that a doctor feels for his patients will make him or her react differently. Lynn's GP's first reaction when she went along to confirm what turned out to be a well-advanced pregnancy, was one of concern: 'My doctor was worried that it was too late even for the tests. That didn't worry me – it wasn't a first-time pregnancy. But it certainly worried him.'

Lynn's doctor expressed his concern throughout her pregnancy – something which Lynn found hard to take: 'I do think my doctor was wrong to appear so worried. When he said it was "too late even for the tests" I knew what he was referring to.'

Fortunately, Lynn herself did not feel worried about the pregnancy although she knew that women who get pregnant later, and certainly women who get pregnant over 40, do run risks of having a handicapped baby: 'But I didn't feel older. I was far more concerned about what I would do afterwards – when the baby was born.'

Both Jean's and Lynn's experiences reflect those of other women. Some are conscious of being older, others less so. But when it comes to the reactions of other people or of hospitals, most do not feel singled out for special treatment other than being offered amniocentesis. It comes as a pleasant surprise to many that their age is less of an issue than they thought. They also very soon realize that they are by no means alone – the booking clinic is often a revelation: 'I was astounded at the number of older women there. I went along expecting to feel like a geriatric mother. In fact the "teenies" were in the minority – the average age must have been between 30 and 35.'

In fact, many women find that the attitudes which they may have been expecting are simply not to be found – either among hospital staff or among their own friends and acquaintances. For the most part, this is largely because they themselves are not nearly so unique as they might have expected. There may be some differences in terms of the stage of setting up home they have reached, but if they look around, most find that they have friends or acquaintances of similar age and with small children in common:

There's a range of attitudes, really. If you go along to the mother-and-toddler group, there tends to be an age gap. There you are with your child in your forties. The problem is people's backgrounds. They're all getting the house with the garden. You're on a plateau above that because you've done it. But all my friends of my age have children under five. They all had jobs and started their families in their early thirties.

I suppose that the people I know now are younger than me - the people that I've met around here where we live. But there is also a core of people - Peter's friends as well as mine. They are our age and they have small families: there's one chap who is nearly 50 whose children are five and two. There's another one who's just had another little boy, whose oldest one is four. We know a lot of people who are in the same situation as us - a lot of second marriages - I suppose we know four or five couples who have very young families.

It's a mixture, really. I have friends who have children the same age and friends with older children. I certainly don't feel out of sync. And I have a lot to do with the NCT and there are a lot of women of different ages and stages.

Advantages

While much has been made of the possible difficulties which women who have their children later in life face, there has been little discussion of the social and emotional gains or losses. What are the advantages and disadvantages? Is it the case that older parents are more settled in their life style and less ready to adjust to the needs of a demanding baby? Is the child an intrusion? What other stresses and strains do older parents have to cope with which they find difficult? And what are the relative advantages to the couple, the child and the whole family? Just what are the benefits of being an older parent? It would seem that, as with being a parent

at any age, the responsibility does have its drawbacks. But, overall, the advantages seem to far outweigh the disadvantages.

For many women, confidence in their child-rearing ability is the key advantage to having children when they are older:

I think when I was younger I went through feeling there were things that I should do - I was very hung up about the 'shoulds' and 'shouldn'ts' of life and as I've got older I've worked through that and that's also to Matthew's advantage. I don't think in terms of what he should be doing at different stages of his development and get worried because he's not doing certain things. Matthew is Matthew and he will do things at his own pace... I don't think I could have thought in these terms when I was much younger – I don't think I would have had the self-confidence to think like that.

I personally would have been more influenced by social and family pressures about child-rearing when I was younger. I would have had less confidence in my mothering skills than I have now. For instance, I probably would not have breast-fed for as long. I probably would have gone with the crowd and breast-fed for a few months. I don't really care what people think and I don't think I'm being a bad mother or a worse mother because I do things differently from the way most people do things. (I weaned him when he was 22 months. I would have continued nursing him if it hadn't been that I wanted to get pregnant again and it seemed unlikely that I would do so until he was fully weaned.)

Some women describe themselves as simply more easy-going, more patient and just more relaxed. Women who have had children both in their twenties and then later may be particularly aware of this. A mother of a twenty-year-old and a two-year-old described the difference in her own confidence, when her older daughter was a baby and now:

I don't mind Karen standing at the kitchen sink slopping water or coating the fish. It makes a terrible mess but it is easily cleared up. When Susan was small, whenever she didn't do what I expected I was shattered. If she didn't eat her carrots my day was ruined. Karen was a very difficult child for the first two years but I didn't worry – I didn't go to the doctor as much and was much more confident in my own judgement. I also had more humour – that's just life, I suppose.

This confidence which women describe is often more to do with their own self-awareness than a knowledge of child-rearing as such:

I think I am more in touch with the intuitive side of myself as I bring him up. Certainly I value things like workshops on different aspects of child development. But basically I feel reasonably confident about my own judgement. There have been times when I have questioned myself, when I've felt for instance it wasn't right to leave him to cry all night. A lot of people say that you really have to get to the point of letting them cry if you want them to sleep all night. I can do that now but I could not do it when he was younger. I feel now that there are very few rights and wrongs about child-rearing. It's much more a matter of doing what suits you – getting your own needs fulfilled as well as fulfilling your child's needs. I think that if I was younger, I might have felt a lot of resentment and guilt because I would have felt that I shouldn't be doing certain things that made Matthew unhappy – like going out and leaving him with a baby-sitter.

When I had my first children I wasn't very mature – I didn't know myself well enough. I didn't exactly feel I was missing out by staying at home with the children, but I wasn't confident that I was doing the right thing and my husband wasn't very helpful. Now I feel I've just got much more to give. I'm more mature and I've got a good relationship and Margaret's just the cherry on top.

The reality, then, for many women is that they are well aware that becoming a mother in their thirties was the right choice or the right outcome for them. Being older and therefore more mature is seen as a definite advantage:

I think that I am personally a better mother than I would have been a few years ago in my twenties. Being older, we really wanted a child – he was very much a wanted child and that's probably the case with most older parents. You are more mature. You have gone through more of life's experiences, so I think that probably most women who are older will have more insight and more awareness of how they might change things where they might be mothering in a way that they are not happy about.
I do feel that the child benefits from having older parents. I sometimes feel quite horrified when I see a young couple with a baby. Some of them look so young, and if the child starts playing up and crying, it's no wonder they can't cope, especially if they have no support. I feel the child does benefit from older parents, but I don't think all women take to it and I don't

think it is something to feel guilty about. If I'd had a career rather than a job, that might have changed things for me.

And women who have had children both in their twenties and then much later may see a sharp contrast between their reactions then and now in their attitudes to motherhood:

Twenty years ago I felt I wasn't doing anything important. I was in four walls, vegetating. I don't think that now. Being responsible for a child is a very important job, but you can't tell someone of twenty that. It's just something you have to arrive at. I don't argue with people. I just think, 'I shouldn't like to be you.'

Although fewer men may be ready to admit these sorts of changes, their attitudes are just as likely to change over the years:

I have so much more patience with Emma now than I had with my first two. I didn't see so much of them – I was always out pursuing my career and trying to get on, going to conferences and evening meetings. Now, I've got wherever I was going and it doesn't matter. Now I get to the end of the day and I just want to be home and give her her bath and see her before she goes to bed. It's really the most important thing for me.

And older fathers with a young family may see themselves as particularly fortunate:

Being an older father has its compensations. I went to have dinner with an old friend whose two children were grown up and leaving home; all he had to talk about were retirement plans and moving to a smaller house. I felt that in remarrying and having another family I was really much younger in my attitudes than he was. It was as if I had a whole second life to live – retirement and old age seemed a world away.

Yet, while so many women talk of their confidence to do the job, it does not necessarily follow that they take to motherhood with great ease and that they are serene and composed from the moment of birth; and even if they do, reality soon changes such expectations:

I had expected to be a better mother because I was older. I had a vision of this Madonna-like, patient person who was going to do a wonderful job of bringing up her son. I've realized, as he gets older, that it's not as easy as that and just because I'm older doesn't mean that I'm better. The kind of mother you are – I think it's more to do with your personality – and that's probably more than just age.

Even so, many older mothers do seem to know how they want to bring up their children and what is right for them:

I find I don't shout now. I really used to shout with Susan when she was little and really let off steam. I don't smack Karen – I find that if I tell her to go into her room and to come out when she's going to behave works better. I just feel now that screaming, shouting and smacking don't always get the best results.

But many admit that they do not always live up to their own ideals when it comes to dealing with an assertive two-year-old:

I feel I've come up against bits of my personality – particularly with a two-year-old. It can be very hard, because they can be so difficult, so one-tracked-minded and determined. They need limits and yet you don't want to set up battlegrounds with them. Yet I have found that there have been times when I really have just lost my temper, just kind of flown off the handle – shouted at him and slapped him – although I don't believe in slapping and I'm really having to think about that very hard, really having to control my feelings of anger.

But while self-confidence may be seen as the basis for coping successfully with being a mother, the self-confidence and success gained in one area of life may be seen as a disadvantage for a woman changing her role from that of career woman to full-time mother:

If you have had a successful career and have felt very self-confident and felt very much in control, a little baby comes along and suddenly life isn't like that any more. You don't have the same control and the same feeling that you are doing your job well. You don't know if you are and there can be problems with young babies that can be really worrying. Are they getting enough to eat? Why aren't they sleeping? Why aren't they on a routine? All these things can possibly worry an older mother more, and in some ways they can be harder to deal with.

For many older parents one of the pleasures of having children later in life is that it may be part of a changing life style – settling down and leading a more content and, for some, satisfying way of life:

> We're very happy and content. She goes three times a week to playgroup and that gives me a couple of hours to do things for myself.
>
> I think it will be marvellous to potter about when she goes to school, doing things in the house or the garden. I shall be quite happy doing that for a few years, having worked for so long. I see all my friends, they work all week and weekends and they are very harassed. But then they can have the holidays abroad. But we've had a good six years' kick at the ball – we had our holidays then, I don't really mind not having them now.

We have no desire to go rushing off to discos and things. We are just more content to stay home. We don't have baby-sitting problems or the frustration of not being able to get out that you see in younger ones. We're quite content to stay here at weekends, a lot of our friends seem to want Easter breaks and so on, although I'm not sure what it is they are 'getting away from' – if they go off to a caravan they are still doing the washing and cleaning. I would love a break from housework, but I don't necessarily need a break from home.

If there are frustrations about not getting out, finding baby-sitters and the lack of holidays abroad, they are most often felt when the baby is still very small and very demanding of time and attention. At this stage the drawbacks can be quite significant and traumatic for a couple who have been together for a long time with no children:

> I think if you've been together for a long time with no children, then when you have a baby it is a terrible shock. You're just not used to this invasion of your time and privacy and the fact that you just can't lead the same sort of life, can't go out as much, can't entertain friends as much, not just because of baby-sitting and so on, but because you're so exhausted. Sleep becomes so precious that nothing in the world is worth a late night.'

What many people forget, or perhaps lose sight of at this difficult and tiring stage, is that three-month-olds all too quickly become quite well-socialized three-year-olds. They do begin to sleep through the night, can be left with sitters and, once they start playgroups and nursery schools, they are very soon on the road to independence.

With all our concern about the responsibilities, rights and wrongs of looking after small children, the very positive aspect of what parents gain from their children is sometimes overlooked. Not working and not running an overloaded daily schedule allows women to take life in their own stride and time to enjoy their children:

I have a friend who is doing an Open University course and every time I see her the house is a mess and the kids are making a scene because she is either writing an essay or trying to read something. There doesn't seem to be any joy. What's the point of doing that? She's getting no joy out of the kids and no joy out of her OU course. If I was rushing round the kids would just be a nuisance to me. I need to have time to discuss things with the kids – explain to my daughter about how I feel at the moment. I think that it is important that they can make adult decisions if you do encourage them to understand the reasoning behind things – that's the satisfaction and pleasure I get.

The joy and pleasure, so important now to one woman, was not something she experienced when she had her first child in her early twenties. With a grown-up daughter and a four-year-old, she is very clear now about her hopes for her daughter's future:

I'd like her to be mature enough to be able to cope with her own life before she has to cope with another. Having said that, I did eventually cope with my first. But it's the joy I get from Karen – the sheer pleasure of being with her and the things that we do. It was a chore to me when Susan was young – I just didn't know that you were supposed to enjoy children.

If there is a danger in getting over-involved in children, it may be that older parents are at risk of spoiling a child and perhaps this is something to be guarded against – not always easy if the child is an only one or if a couple have had problems conceiving:

Of course you take a risk in waiting because you don't know that you will become pregnant quite so easily when you are older, and I think that's why, when you do have a child, you treat that child as if that child might be your only one. I don't know whether there is a danger of spoiling the child. It depends what you mean by spoiling. I don't think it is wrong to give a child what it needs in terms of attention and lots of affection, but to overindulge is spoiling.

Finally, there is the question of how the child with older parents will get on as he or she gets older. Will this be a disadvantage? Is he or she likely to be isolated in this respect? Even though this may be an issue which worries some older parents, with current trends and the likelihood of more babies being born to older parents in the next few years, it will probably become irrelevant – as one woman observed: 'I think there are going to be enough other children with older parents that it doesn't necessarily need to be an issue, particularly as there are plenty of people who have their youngest child when they are older – so there will be plenty of children with older parents.'

CHAPTER TWO

Pregnancy and Looking After Yourself

Many women who have spent some time considering pregnancy want to make sure that they are in the best of health and have done everything possible to ensure they have a healthy child. There are some practical steps which you can take in advance to prepare yourself for the healthiest possible pregnancy.

Stopping contraception

If you have been relying on an IUD, you will need to have it removed by a doctor before you conceive. If you get pregnant by chance with an IUD in place it does carry risks for mother and baby. You are more likely to have an ectopic pregnancy – a pregnancy which occurs outside the womb, usually in the fallopian tubes – and there is a high risk of miscarriage for a pregnancy with an IUD in place. As many as 60 per cent of such pregnancies end before term, and these miscarriages are also more likely to occur in the second three months of pregnancy.

As soon as an IUD is removed, you can get pregnant. IUDs are usually removed while you have a period, as the cervix is then slightly dilated and this aids removal.

If you have been taking the contraceptive pill, it is now advised that you stop taking it for two or three months before you wish to conceive. You can use a barrier method such as the sheath or diaphragm or natural family planning (rhythm method) during this time, although you are unlikely to use natural family planning effectively if you have not spent some time learning the technique and observing your menstrual cycle. Studies have shown that women who have taken the pill inadvertently in early pregnancy are in fact running only the very slightest extra risk of having an abnormal baby or pregnancy, and that those who conceive as soon as they stop the pill face no extra risk. But it is a wise precaution to make sure that your body is free of all drugs before you get pregnant. It also helps to date the pregnancy if you have had one or two normal menstrual cycles before you conceive and allows for good pregnancy care.

There is, however, some evidence that women who conceive while using spermicides, whether on their own or in combination with the diaphragm or cap or sheath, run a slightly increased risk of having a miscarriage (and, incidentally, also a greater chance of having a girl). It is obviously better to conceive when there are no traces of spermicide in the vagina.

If you intend to try to conceive, it may be a good idea to ask your GP to do a cervical smear and perhaps to take a swab to check that you do not have any vaginal infection such as thrush before you get pregnant. This will usually be done at your first hospital appointment when you are pregnant, anyway, but some women prefer not to have a vaginal examination in early pregnancy, especially if they have had a miscarriage or threatened miscarriage in the past. It also makes sense to clear up any infection before rather than after a pregnancy has begun.

Avoiding drugs in pregnancy

Many women are aware that taking any drugs – including tobacco and alcohol – during pregnancy can have a harmful effect on the growing and developing baby. This is especially important in the first three months, when the baby is actually forming, as this is the time when any abnormalities would occur. Women and their partners who are planning a pregnancy, then, need to think about giving up smoking and cutting down drinking, ensuring that their diet contains all the elements necessary for the baby's healthy growth, and stopping any unnecessary medication. Any woman taking drugs essential for her health (for diabetes, epilepsy or high blood pressure, for example), should discuss this matter very carefully with her doctor.

There is some evidence that heavy smoking or drinking on the part of the father before conception can affect the quantity and quality of his sperm, and some drugs may also affect sperm production, so some men may need to think about this too. Sperm production takes about three months, so the father should also be thinking about changing some of his habits three or four months before you plan to get pregnant.

Alcohol

There has been a lot of controversy about the effect of taking alcohol during pregnancy, and a number of studies have been done. There is now no doubt that heavy drinking in pregnancy can have very serious effects on the baby, at its worst causing what is known as the foetal alcohol syndrome. Such babies have low birth-weight, and do not catch up as do the babies of malnourished mothers or babies who have not been receiving enough nourishment in the womb. Their head circumference is smaller, and there is often mental retardation. Some have odd facial characteristics and there is a higher incidence of congenital heart disease and other abnormalities. The greater the level of alcohol drunk by the mother, the more severe the abnormalities are likely to be, and the greater the risk of the baby being miscarried or stillborn.

The situation for mothers who are moderate social drinkers is less clear, although there does appear to be evidence that women who do not drink at all in pregnancy are less likely to have miscarriages or low-birth-weight babies. However, the first three months appear to be the crucial time, during which the abnormalities associated with the foetal alcohol syndrome may occur. Doctors and health experts are now advising that women do not drink at all in pregnancy, and probably the best thing is to give up all alcohol when you are trying to conceive and not drink at all in the first three to four months of pregnancy, or indeed for the whole nine months.

Cigarettes

Smoking in pregnancy is very clearly linked to a higher risk of miscarriage and to low birth-weight. There is no evidence to link congenital abnormalities with smoking, although the risk of the baby being stillborn or dying in the first few weeks of life is definitely greater, and babies are much more likely to be born prematurely.

If you are a smoker, the best time to stop is before you get pregnant. However, giving up is not necessarily that easy. Women who smoke do so for reasons which are important to them. Some women say it helps them to relax, others that it keeps their weight down. Many women find that the best way to give up smoking is to substitute something else in its place. If you smoke to relieve stress,

you can try yoga for relaxation, or some other form of exercise. If your weight is really a problem, make sure that you read all the advice about the importance of diet in pregnancy. Following this should make sure you do not gain any unnecessary pounds. If your partner smokes, try and stop together – his moral support will boost your will-power and set the scene for a smoke-free household when the baby does arrive. Or find a friend who also wants to stop smoking and give each other positive support.

Painkillers

Aspirin

Aspirin is probably the most commonly used of all drugs, and in fact its use is so common that many people do not take it seriously as a drug at all. Aspirin is known to cross the placenta into the baby's bloodstream, but its effects on the baby are not really known. Some studies, however, have shown that aspirin in large quantities may increase the risk of miscarriage in the first three months and have other harmful effects later on, so you should use aspirin sparingly in pregnancy.

Paracetamol

Paracetamol is known to affect the liver and kidneys if taken in large quantities and could affect the developing foetus, so again should be used only sparingly in pregnancy.

Tranquillizers

There has been evidence that some tranquillizers cause an increase in birth defects, notably in cleft lip and palate.

The evidence is not clear, but wherever possible tranquillizers should be avoided during pregnancy, especially in the first three months.

Antibiotics

Some antibiotics are known to be safe in pregnancy; others are definitely harmful. Penicillin is thought to be safe; tetracycline causes yellow discolouration of the baby's teeth and may affect the growth of bones and teeth; streptomycin may be linked to deafness. You should always make sure any doctor prescribing antibiotics for you is aware that you are pregnant.

Hormonal drugs

The evidence shows that women who have taken the contraceptive pill inadvertently early in pregnancy are not at any substantial risk of affecting the baby; women who used post-coital hormonal contraception which failed also do not seem to be at risk. Other hormonal drugs given early in pregnancy, however, do have very definite harmful effects. Hormones given in some kinds of pregnancy tests (now withdrawn from the market) caused baby girls to develop male characteristics. A drug called DES (diethylstilboestrol), given early in pregnancy to prevent miscarriage is now know to be linked to a rare vaginal cancer in babies born to these mothers, together with some abnormalities of the internal sex organs. Other hormones, such as progestogens, given in pregnancy to prevent miscarriage or for other problems, may have harmful effects and are best avoided, although there is no conclusive evidence to prove

this. In some cases where a woman has miscarried because of low hormone levels, this treatment may be justified.

Anti-nausea drugs

The use of anti-nausea drugs in pregnancy is very controversial. Thalidomide was given to women to prevent sickness in early pregnancy and shocked the world by the horrific abnormalities it caused. Other drugs have been used to prevent nausea and vomiting in the first three months of pregnancy, but most of these have also been eventually withdrawn because of a possible link with birth defects (Debendox is one).

Because the baby is so very vulnerable to drugs in the first three months of pregnancy when nausea occurs, taking any kind of drug must be viewed as a last resort, and anyone who can possibly manage without drugs would be well advised to. However, getting the support to do so may not be easy.

I had terrible nausea and vomiting in both my pregnancies. In the second pregnancy it was worse, and lasted from five weeks (that was how I knew I was pregnant) to 16. I felt sick every minute of the day, and I was sick frequently – two or three times some days, only once on others. It wasn't just in the morning, it was all or anytime, and was worse when I didn't eat regular, small snacks and meals. At around seven or eight weeks I had 48 hours when I couldn't keep anything down, and because I had an active toddler to look after, I was getting desperate. I rang the doctor who suggested an antinausea drug, and I said "no". In fact, the vomiting did get better after that acute phase and I did manage to eat, though I lost weight over the first three months. After sixteen weeks it got dramatically better, and I was so pleased that I got through without drugs. I know I would have been worried sick for the rest of the pregnancy that there'd be something wrong with the baby if I'd taken anything. I wish doctors would help give you confidence to go without drugs unless you really can't keep anything down at all.'

But some women do experience such severe nausea that they are only able to get through this phase with the help of medication:

I was expecting twin boys and I was so sick I couldn't even keep down a glass of water, so in the end I took Debendox (this was before it was withdrawn). There was nothing wrong with the twins at all, they are fantastic, perfect. I just couldn't have carried on without.

There are, however, alternatives to drugs, including herbal drinks or homoeo-pathic remedies which some women find help with nausea and vomiting. But the best way to cope with nausea and vomiting seems to be careful attention to diet, which should consist of nutritious foods such as wholemeal bread, fresh fruit, nuts, raisins and dried fruit, raw vegetables; cereals; wholemeal biscuits and muesli bars can be good if you want something sweet. Eating small, frequent amounts helps. Fatty or very sweet foods are likely to make you feel worse rather than better, and you should avoid spicy food, alcohol, or cigarette smoke. If preparing food makes you feel ill, get someone else to do it for you if at all possible, or have meals that need the minimum preparation. Drink plenty of (mainly fresh) fruit juices, herbal teas and water; avoid tea and coffee – and many people find milky drinks make sickness worse, too. Remember to keep on eating regardless. It is much more unpleasant being sick on an empty stomach than a full one, and starving yourself is likely to make the nausea much worse. Even if food stays in the stomach only a short time, some goodness will have been absorbed.

Diet during pregnancy

Maintaining a healthy diet during pregnancy is the best thing you can do for yourself and for your baby. If you eat the right foods, you won't need to worry about taking vitamin supplements and you won't need to worry about whether you're putting on the right amount of weight or not; your body will do that automatically.

Weight gain
It is normal to gain weight in pregnancy.

Most of this weight is put on in the second three months of pregnancy. The increased weight will be the weight of the baby, the placenta, the waters surrounding the baby, increased fluid and tissue in the breasts as they prepare to produce milk, and a greater quantity of blood circulating in the body. Some women also experience fluid retention which will adjust after the baby is born. So it's quite wrong to think that all the additional weight apart from the baby is fat – it isn't!

A normal weight gain is 20–30 lbs (9–13.5 kg) during pregnancy. Some women gain less, others more, without there being any need for alarm. If you are planning to breast-feed your baby, you should also remember that you will be laying down some stores of fat to feed your new baby and that the pounds will roll off as you produce your milk. Doctors used to worry a lot about 'excessive' weight gain in pregnancy as this can put an extra strain on the body, making high blood pressure and cardio-vascular problems more likely. However, this in itself was a reaction to the exhortations previously made to women to 'eat for two'. But aiming for the other extreme and trying to stay slim in pregnancy is equally harmful. It is particularly damaging to try to 'diet' in pregnancy as you may be denying the baby vital nourishment. Again, eating the right food is the key. If you eat well you will feel well, be less inclined to want to 'fill up' on sweet things, and your body will gain and shed weight naturally during and after the pregnancy.

A healthy diet

A healthy diet means eating a balanced combination of proteins, carbohydrates, fats, and vitamins. This can be achieved by eating reasonable quantities of fresh meat and fish, eggs, cheese and milk, fresh fruits and vegetables, wholemeal bread and cereals. Avoid foods which have 'empty' calories, such as highly refined sugary cakes and sweet fizzy drinks, biscuits, salty foods which will encourage fluid retention, and drinks like coffee, tea and cocoa, as well as wine, spirits and beer.

What you need and why

Protein

Proteins contain the basic building blocks that make up your body and are absolutely vital in pregnancy for the baby to grow and develop. Your protein requirements go up by about 50 per cent during pregnancy. The best sources of protein are in meat and fish, dairy products, eggs and in pulses and some green vegetables – lentils, peas, beans, seeds, nuts and yeast are all very rich in protein. If you are a vegetarian you can still get enough protein from the latter, but some vegetarian women prefer to eat a little fish and chicken in pregnancy to boost their protein intake. Fish is particularly valuable, as it contains a lot of minerals and vitamins and is also low in fat.

Carbohydrates

Carbohydrates are vital in meeting your energy needs in pregnancy. They do not have to be fattening: Potatoes, especially if baked in their jackets, are not fattening and also contain a lot of vitamin C. Bread, flour, cereals and root vegetables are all good sources of carbohydrate, and it's best not to skip these; you may then feel hungry again and fill up on sweet things instead.

Fat

You do not need extra fat in pregnancy, and if you are gaining excessive weight you can cut down on butter, oils and sauces and have low-fat yogurts and curd cheese. However, you will need to make sure you are not missing out on the fat-soluble vitamins.

Minerals

A number of minerals are known to be essential for health, and especially during pregnancy. Because the body's blood volume increases so much, there is an extra demand for iron in pregnancy, and this is especially true in second and subsequent pregnancies, especially if there has not been a long gap since the last baby was born. You can increase iron in the blood by eating iron-rich foods, notably dark green vegetables such as spinach and watercress, offal such as liver and kidneys, egg yolks, whole grains, pulses and nuts. Your haemoglobin levels will be checked in pregnancy to make sure that you are not getting anaemic; if you are, iron pills can be prescribed.

Calcium is important in pregnancy for the formation of bones and teeth and to ensure blood-clotting. Milk and dairy foods are a good source, but so are vegetables, whole grains, pulses and nuts. Spinach, rhubarb and cocoa help prevent the absorption of calcium, so do not have too much of these foods.

Potassium, zinc and other trace elements are also important. Seafood is a good source of many minerals and oysters are particularly rich in zinc!

Fibre

Many women find that they tend to become constipated in pregnancy, as the pregnancy hormones slow down the movement of the muscles of the bowel. Constipation can make mothers feel unwell, as well as leading to piles if you are constantly straining on the loo. It is important to eat foods which have plenty of fibre – wholemeal bread, unrefined cereals like muesli or those which are rich in bran, and raw fruit and vegetables. It is important to drink a lot of fluids.

Vitamins

Vitamins are essential in pregnancy, both to keep you healthy and for the development of your baby. Research has shown that mothers who are short of certain vitamins are at a greater risk of having a handicapped baby or a baby who is born with low birth-weight. Table 2 shows what vitamins you need and what they do.

Since a pregnancy is not usually confirmed till six or eight weeks, and it may take a little time for the body to build up depleted stores of vitamins and essential minerals, it is very important to adjust your diet before you become pregnant if at all possible. A good diet will also make you feel stronger and healthier and help you through the demanding months of pregnancy, through the birth itself, and through the post-natal period. It will help you to enjoy your baby, too.

Table 2   Essential nutrients during pregnancy

Nutrient	Rich sources	Good sources	What it does
Vitamin A	Egg yolk, oily fish, whole milk, butter, carrots	Liver, kidneys, green and yellow vegetables	Helps resist infection, essential for vision, keeps hair etc. in good condition.
Vitamin B1 Thiamine	Wheatgerm, nuts, pork	Oatmeal, liver, kidney, peas, wholemeal bread	Aids digestion, necessary for growth.
Vitamin B2 Riboflavin	Brewer's yeast, wheatgerm	Green vegetables, milk, eggs, liver	Builds brain cells, prevents infections and bleeding gums.
Niacin	Beef extract, liver, peanuts, salmon, sardines	Kidney, cooked meats, mackerel, other fish	Prevents eye and and skin problems, essential for normal growth and de-velopment.
Vitamin B6 Pyridoxine	Yeast, liver kidney, mackerel	Meat, fish, eggs, banana, pineapple, wholemeal bread	Deficiency causes disease of the nerves and anaemia.
Vitamin B12	Liver, pilchards, sardines, herring	Tongue, turkey, tuna, salmon, beef, lamb, egg	Necessary to form red blood cells and nervous system.
Folic acid	Liver, dark green vegetables	Kidney, peanuts, walnuts, wheatgerm, eggs, lettuce, mushroom, tomatoes, oranges	As above. Deficiency linked to spina bifida.
Vitamin C Ascorbic acid	Blackcurrants, strawberries broccoli, sprouts, cabbage	oranges, lemons, broad beans, asparagus	Helps iron absorption, im-portant for healing.

Nutrient	Rich sources	Good sources	What it does
Calcium	Milk, hard cheese	Small whole fish, especially shellfish, soya flour, figs, peanuts, walnuts	Essential for healthy bones and teeth.
Iron	Liver, black sausage, kidney, beef, soya, oysters	Lamb, chicken, turkey, ham	Essential for formation of red blood cells.
Zinc	Oysters, wheat-germ, wheat bran	Beef, lamb, liver, cheese, milk, oatmeal, whole-grain cereals	Helps form many enzymes and proteins.

Preconceptual care

As the idea of preconceptual care becomes more widely known, more and more mothers are trying to prepare well in advance for the birth of their baby. Genetic counsellors are available through the NHS if there is any genetic disorder in the family or if you are at greater risk of having a handicapped baby. Advice on diet and general health care in pregnancy may be given at your antenatal clinic.

There is an organization, Foresight, which gives information and advice to women who are planning a pregnancy. Foresight will also do tests of samples of your hair and blood to check that you are well nourished and not short of any essential vitamins or minerals. However, many doctors believe that this is unrealistic, and that in most cases the shortage of vitamins and minerals would not be enough to place the mother at higher risk of having an abnormal baby. It is also true that the majority of women do not want to wait months to conceive, and many conceive by accident, or experience problems in conceiving, and these mothers may feel guilty that they are not doing the right thing:

We started out with all the best intentions, stopping smoking and drinking, taking vitamin pills and potions and eating only health-foody things without any additives. But it took me nearly two years to get pregnant. By the end I was fed up with the whole thing – we never enjoyed ourselves any more, we felt guilty about everything we ate or didn't eat. In the end I just ate what I felt like and got on with it.

Foresight also provides genetic counselling for those who are worried that they may be at extra risk of having a handicapped baby – this includes older mothers and those who have some hereditary illness or defect in their family. Genetic counselling is also available at many hospitals:

> We had genetic counselling at the hospital because I was 40, my husband was in his forties too, and his child by his previous marriage had had problems – her gullet and windpipe were joined and there was a blockage to the entrance to her stomach. She had to be operated on at birth, although she's fine now. We were told that this could be picked up on the ultrasound scan, as the baby would not be able to swallow the amniotic fluid which would otherwise show up in the stomach – this was very reassuring as we would want to know in advance so the baby could be born where they would be geared up to do immediate surgery. I was also concerned about the extra risk of having a Down's Syndrome baby – I was surprised at how greatly the risk went up between the ages of 40 and 41. We decided to have the amnio-

centesis and other tests done because we felt we couldn't have coped with a severely handicapped baby. I found the counselling very helpful and reassuring.

Genetic counselling can be very helpful in enabling the couple to talk through any worries they have and to put the risks they are facing into proportion. It can also be very helpful in establishing the reasons for any previous babies born with handicaps in the family, or for several miscarriages, and point towards ways of overcoming them. For example, it has been shown that mothers of babies with spina bifida had far fewer affected babies in subsequent pregnancies if they took supplements of vitamin B and folic acid. Some couples who have had several miscarriages have been told that this is linked to a genetic problem but that if they persist there is a chance they will have a normal baby, and this has encouraged them to carry on.

Keeping fit in pregnancy

Exercise and general physical fitness are very important in pregnancy. Your body changes shape and new stresses and strains are put on it, culminating in the physical stress of the birth itself. By making sure your body is strong and fit you will be helping yourself in pregnancy and working towards an active and safe birth, as well as giving yourself energy and resilience for the demanding time ahead.

During pregnancy your joints tend to loosen slightly; this enables the pelvis to stretch during birth to let the baby through, but also means that you are more likely to strain your ligaments and joints and, especially, your back. You should be careful of putting strain on your back by picking things up awkwardly or carrying loads which are too heavy. The weight of your baby in front will make even simple movements like getting out of a chair or bed potentially damaging for your back, so take care to move in such a way as not to put undue strain on it. Roll over onto your side and sit up from there to get out of bed and use your legs, not your back, to lever

Lifting heavy weights:

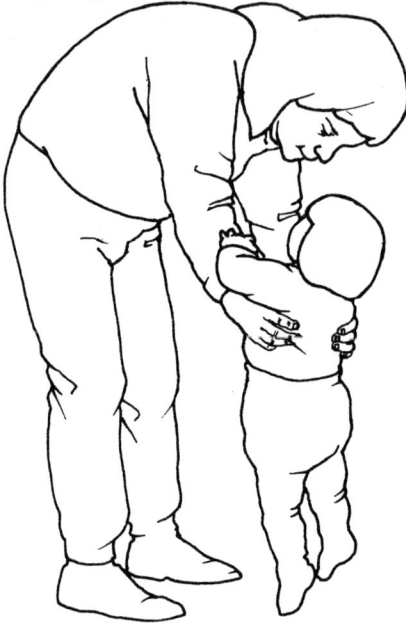 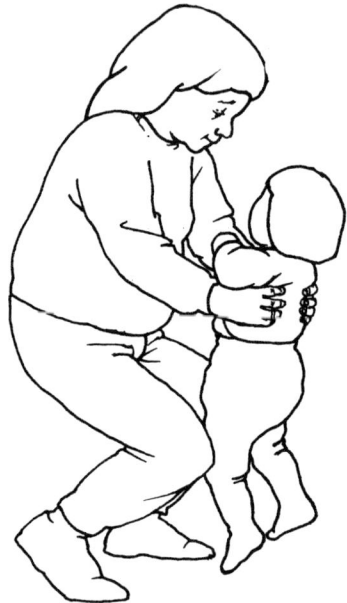

wrong   right

yourself out of a chair. When picking up a toddler or bag of shopping, squat down and then push up with your thighs rather than bending your back right over.

There are a number of exercises you can do in pregnancy to keep yourself supple and to strengthen muscles that you will use in the birth itself. However, not everyone is very good at doing a programme of exercises and if you are working, or you have other children, it may be hard to fit them in. Gentle walking and, especially, swimming are good exercises in pregnancy if you enjoy them. You can carry on with your usual

sports, but remember that if you get out of breath you are depriving your baby of oxygen too. Exercise in pregnancy should be gentle rather than fierce.

Women who want an active labour should practise holding positions such as squatting, standing on all fours or sitting in a semi-upright position to see what position they find most comfortable and to strengthen the muscles they will use. All women, however, will benefit from locating and exercising the pelvic floor muscles which are so important in pregnancy and childbirth. These muscles support the uterus, bowel and bladder and about half of all women who have had children suffer from some weakness in these muscles, with such symptoms as discomfort in the pelvic area or leaking a little urine when they sneeze, cough or lift heavy objects. If these muscles become too weak it can lead to prolapse of the womb.

You can feel what it is like to use the pelvic floor muscles by tightening your buttocks and pulling upwards as if you want to empty your bladder but must hold on. The same muscle tightens the vagina and can cause pleasant sensations when you are making love. If you cannot feel the muscles tighten, then try interrupting the flow of urine when you are emptying your bladder; you will soon be able to recognize the sensation of tensing these muscles.

You can exercise these muscles unseen every day when you are lying down, standing or sitting. Simply do four to six contractions of about five seconds each at various intervals during the day. You can try to do them at the same times each day – when you're cleaning your teeth or in the bath, washing up, and so on – to help you incorporate them in your daily routine. It is important to carry on with these exercises after the baby is born, to strengthen them after the inevitable stretching they will have received during the birth.

Antenatal care

Good antenatal care, as well as taking care of your health and looking after yourself, is the key to a healthy pregnancy, and doctors and other health professionals are aware that it is only through improving antenatal care that they can improve the health of mothers and babies and reduce the small number of babies who are born with difficulties and who die. Much of the antenatal care you will receive is routine, but it is there to pick up any problems and take action to prevent them from getting worse. Skipping on appointments or failing to make use of the services available is putting yourself and your baby at risk, and this may be particularly so for the older mother.

Finding out you are pregnant

Most women will want to know that they are pregnant as soon as possible, especially if they have had problems conceiving. There are now modern pregnancy tests available which can tell you accurately whether you are pregnant or not as soon as your period is due. These tests are available from chemists at a modest price – each packet usually contains two tests, so that if the first isn't positive, you can repeat it a few days later to make sure. Because these tests are rather more expensive than the standard test carried out by your doctor two weeks after your first missed period, they are not usually available on the

NHS. You will find that if you get a pregnancy test done free through your GP, hospital or family-planning clinic, it will not usually be done earlier than when your period is two weeks overdue and that you will not usually have to wait for the result.

> It was silly because when my period was overdue I did a home test and it was positive. Then they did one at Bart's [St Bartholomew's Hospital, London] and it was negative. We were both very disappointed. But my period didn't start, and I *felt* pregnant. So I did another home test which was positive. I rang my husband and asked him to pop home from work and check I wasn't imagining it, and he agreed it was positive. But the next test from the hospital was negative too – until the GP rang and said they had made an error.
>
> It seemed so silly that a home test was so much better than the hospital one!

Having your pregnancy confirmed early enables you to stop drinking, take care of your diet, if you haven't already done so, and book early for your antenatal appointments. Once you know you are pregnant you should talk things over with your GP and explain any preferences you have for the kind of birth you would like, which hospitals you prefer, whether you would like a GP delivery if possible and whether you would like a home birth if that can be arranged. Your GP will know the options in the area and will be able to discuss with you what is best, and then may refer you to the system of your choice. In practice this is not always the case, and older mothers in particular may find they are only offered a hospital birth or are under strong pressure to have the baby in hospital. In some areas, too, the choice of hospital is limited. Many GPs do not do deliveries at all.

The vast majority of births now take place in hospitals and most people also have their antenatal care under the hospital. Even if you are having a hospital birth, however, you can arrange to have shared care with your GP, if he or she does obstetric care, which may mean shorter waits for appointments as well as the comfort of a familiar face. You may also be seen by a midwife at your doctor's surgery, especially if it is part of a larger health clinic. Although things seem to have improved in antenatal care, the majority of women find waiting at the hospital clinics is still a problem. There are usually no facilities for older children and toddlers. Women complain that they are seen by someone different each time and never even see the consultant they are booked under, and many women find the care impersonal and offhand. If you have any special problems, you are more likely to see the consultant, so if you just see the midwife at every visit you can console yourself with the fact that your pregnancy is progressing normally.

On the whole, older mothers do not find themselves too much of an oddity at antenatal clinics:

> I realized that I could be the mother of the women sitting next to me, but it didn't really seem to matter. We were both going through the same thing. I

was never once made to feel by the other women or by the hospital staff that I was old or doing anything out the ordinary.

I should think the average age of mothers at the hospital was 30–35, though this hospital does specialize in women with potential difficulties and older mothers and it is London, which I think makes a difference. I was astounded at the number of older women – it seems women have their careers first and then their families.

Routine antenatal tests

You are usually booked for your first appointment at around the twelfth week of pregnancy, when your medical history will be taken, together with any details of previous pregnancies. Your height and shoe size are measured, as this gives some indication of the size of your pelvis, though women usually have babies in proportion to their own size. You are also likely to be given an internal examination to confirm the pregnancy and check the womb is the size it should be for your dates, check for any abnormalities of the pelvis and check that the cervix (neck of the womb) is tightly closed. A cervical smear is also taken. If you have had a history of miscarriage it is likely that the doctor will agree not to examine you at this stage if you wish, though there is no particular evidence to suggest that this might provoke a miscarriage. You are also screened for any sexually transmitted disease.

At every visit you will be weighed to check the growth of the baby and that your weight gain is satisfactory. Your urine is tested at every visit – the first time it will be screened for any infection, every other visit it will be tested for the presence of protein in the urine which could indicate you have pre-eclampsia (see below). The abdomen is measured at every visit to check that the womb is growing in size according to your dates and after 20–24 weeks your baby's heartbeat can be monitored with a stethoscope or sometimes a device called a sonic-aid. Your blood pressure is also measured at every visit, as high blood pressure can indicate a number of problems including pre-eclampsia, and your ankles and fingers are checked for water retention.

A number of blood tests are carried out at your first visit to determine your blood group, whether you are immune to the German measles (rubella) virus, and to detect various diseases, including syphilis, which must be treated before giving birth. Your blood will also be tested for haemoglobin levels early and later in the pregnancy to check that you are not anaemic.

Pre-eclampsia or toxaemia is one condition that doctors are on the alert for in pregnancy, as it can be prevented if caught early and the risk to the unborn baby be reduced. Older mothers are at a greater risk of this condition, so it's important to keep up regular visits. The cause is unknown, although in some cases it has been linked to poor nutrition. The symptoms are water retention, causing puffiness of ankles, legs and wrists, high blood pressure, and if the condition is allowed to progress unchecked, blood pressure rises further, the mother suffers headaches and even fits. The baby is at risk and may not be getting enough nourishment, and there is an increased risk of premature labour.

Pre-eclampsia can usually be treated by bed rest, and women suffering this condition are often admitted to hospital so that they and the baby can be monitored. Usually complete rest solves the problem, but if it does get worse, the baby may have to be born early by Caesarian section to ensure that it survives.

Twin pregnancies

It may come as a surprise to learn that older mothers are more likely to have twins than their younger counterparts. Identical twins are the result of the fertilized egg splitting in two and developing in exactly the same way, since they contain exactly the same genetic material. This occurs at random and does not seem to be influenced by heredity or age. Non-identical twins occur when two eggs are released in a cycle by the ovary, and are both fertilized. Non-identical twins are no more alike than other brothers and sisters, and the chance of having them increases with age, and especially if there are other non-identical twins in the family or if a woman has been taking certain fertility drugs to conceive.

A twin pregnancy needs special care and monitoring as it puts an extra strain on your body. You will need to watch for high blood pressure and anaemia and will need extra rest. Twin babies are more likely to be born prematurely and sometimes one baby grows larger than the other, which may be of low birthweight – or both babies may be underweight. The birth will need to take place in hospital as there is an increased risk to the second baby if it is not born soon after the first, especially if it is not in the usual head-down position.

Emotional changes in pregnancy

It is as important to take care of yourself emotionally in pregnancy as it is to take care of your physical well-being, although this is much more difficult. Many women find that they change a lot in pregnancy, that they feel more vulnerable and easily upset, or that they become preoccupied with the new life inside them and find it more difficult to keep up at work, to visit friends or to put energy into making their relationship with their partner run smoothly. Pregnancy can thus be a very testing time for many couples, though potentially a very rewarding one, too.

A woman's feelings may depend on how well she feels in pregnancy as well as on the closeness of her relationships with partner, family and friends and, perhaps most important of all, how much the pregnancy was planned and hoped for.

I got pregnant by accident – I wasn't too pleased when I got the news! I had a teenage daughter by my first marriage and none in my second, but we'd agreed not to have any. My initial reaction was resentment and the doctor offered a termination – I woke up and cried every morning to think that I was pregnant. But my husband had no children in his first marriage and when I sat and thought about an abortion I couldn't have done it because of him.

After infertility tests and a miscarriage I was so thrilled to be pregnant that I went around in a haze for the whole pregnancy, despite morning sickness and other discomforts. I couldn't contain myself, it was so exciting.

Some women find work becomes a strain:

It was difficult staggering into work in the early months with bad morning sickness. I used to throw up regularly in the office loo as soon as I got in – the miracle was I was never sick on the bus!

Then, later, I used to sit at meetings and be unable to concentrate properly because the baby was kicking so much – it seemed so odd to be there talking about work plans and schedules while this tremendous thing was going on inside me. I also became very cow-like and contented – I couldn't rush for deadlines any more, they seemed so unimportant.

Others find that they can really relax and enjoy the pregnancy and live it to the full: 'I felt great when pregnant. I relaxed

and let myself be taken care of.'

A great deal has been written about post-natal depression, but very little about antenatal depression, although it is quite common for women to be depressed in some stages of pregnancy. Many women feel overwhelmingly tired and this means that social engagements, work, housework and relationships all suffer if people do not understand:

I used to go to bed whenever I could so the house got in a terrible mess because I couldn't face cleaning it. I couldn't be bothered to cook nice meals and I didn't have the energy to go out to parties or the cinema with friends. My husband used to groan because every evening about nine o'clock I'd just say, I'm exhausted, I'm going to bed now. A lot of the time I was too tired for sex as well.

Depression is perhaps particularly common in a second pregnancy, especially when the woman has a toddler or young child to care for, and/or is working. No one makes quite the same fuss of you after the first pregnancy and it is harder to get the extra rest you need. Again, working women may find pregnancy particularly tiring and feel that they are not being so efficient in their jobs, which again can cause feelings of depression.

Older women in pregnancy may worry about the health of their baby and about the birth itself – whether they will have complications and whether there will be anything wrong with the baby. This may also depend on the attitude of the doctors and midwives caring for the woman in pregnancy:

I found out I was pregnant in my early forties by accident too late to have an abortion or even the tests – my GP was very nervous about it all and my husband worried and thought something would be wrong. The scans gave a different date to my GP and said the baby was small – it was all a worry.

I worried about the birth because of my age, but the consultant was fantastic. He said, 'You're a healthy woman – you should have a super easy birth' – he was very reassuring.

Sex in pregnancy

Many couples continue with a happy and fulfilling sex life right through the pregnancy, and doctors today reassure women that sex in pregnancy is perfectly safe and will not harm the baby. There are a few circumstances in which this is not so: women who have had a history of miscarriage or threatened miscarriage may be advised to avoid sexual intercourse until after the time when the miscarriage or threat occurred, or till after the first 12–16 weeks of pregnancy. Women who have had a premature labour may also be advised to avoid intercourse in the last months, for fear of precipitating labour. In a normal pregnancy, however, there is no evidence that having sexual intercourse or experiencing an orgasm will upset the pregnancy.

Many women find that they get increased pleasure from sex in pregnancy; the increased blood supply to the genital area and the strong contractions of the womb during orgasm can all heighten sensation. Some women feel a particular closeness to their partners in pregnancy which they need to express sexually and others seek reassurance that they are still desirable.

Not all women feel this, however, and some feel that they need to retreat somewhat into their bodies and concentrate on the baby, and that sex is an intrusion into this. Tiredness and other discomforts at the end of pregnancy may also make some women feel less like sex, while some may feel that other ways of expressing love and affection are more appropriate. One small study into women's feelings about sex before and after the birth showed that only half the women in the sample were still having sexual intercourse twelve weeks before the birth, so these feelings are very normal.

Towards the end of pregnancy, sex in the usual positions may become very uncomfortable so it is a good idea to experiment with other positions – something which many couples also find adds to their sex life. A lot of women find full penetration very uncomfortable at the end of pregnancy, especially when the baby's head has 'engaged' and dropped right down into the pelvis, so positions which avoid too deep penetration are preferable. It is important for women to talk openly to their partners about their wishes and feelings in pregnancy; otherwise sex can become a focus for dissatisfaction and resentment.

CHAPTER THREE

Still Not Pregnant

Am I fertile?

If you have decided to go ahead and have a baby, you may now be asking yourself how long will it in fact take for you to get pregnant. There is no straightforward answer to this question. Some people seem to get pregnant very easily, while some take several months or longer to conceive. Some couples have problems getting pregnant at all and only do so after medical treatment.

Fertility in women does begin to fall after the age of 25, but the decline is very slow and it is not until a woman reaches the age of 35 that it is very significant. After that, fertility begins to fall quite rapidly. On the other hand, in some women there appears to be a sudden increase in fertility in women around the age of 39 which, it is claimed, is the reason why some women with grown-up families find themselves pregnant. This is sometimes referred to as the 'last fling of the ovaries'.

Women are usually so concerned with the need to avoid pregnancy that it is hardly surprising that most simply assume that they will get pregnant as soon as they stop using contraception. It may come as something of a shock when this does not happen: 'It's such a joke that for years and years you're taking the pill or whatever and you decide to get pregnant – three years later you're still not pregnant! It's a real shock. That's what happened to us.'

As each month passes and your period comes again, you may begin to think that your chances of getting pregnant are not that great. And if you have waited to have your baby you may be panicking at the thought that time is passing. No one can say what an individual's chances of getting pregnant are, but the overall picture gives some indications of what might happen. First of all, it may be helpful to know that it is perfectly normal to have to wait several months; long-term studies show that 50 per cent of women who are trying to get pregnant do so within six months. It will take 40 per cent between six months and a year. But one in ten will have difficulty in achieving a pregnancy.

The chance of pregnancy is dependent on a number of conditions being just right. You have to produce an egg from one or other of the ovaries. The egg develops each month under control of hormones from the brain. In the early part of the cycle, the ovary produces the hormone oestrogen. This helps the growth and release of an egg from the ovary (ovulation). As the egg matures, the lining of the uterus (womb) changes in case you get pregnant. (Oestrogen also encourages the production of cervical mucus and most women are aware of how this varies throughout the cycle.) A man must be producing enough sperm. The sperms are produced in the testes or testicles and there are many millions – in each ejaculation up to 300,000 million sperm are deposited in the vagina. They travel through the tubes called the vas deferens and the urethra and are released from the penis when the man ejaculates. The sperms have to be able to get inside the vagina to reach the cervix which is the entrance to the uterus (womb), and then through the uterus to the fallopian tubes where fertilization takes place. If an egg

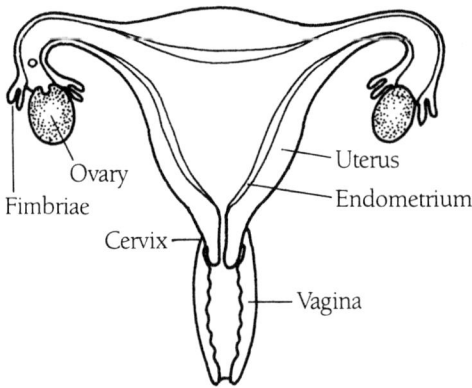

1 Egg is released from ovary

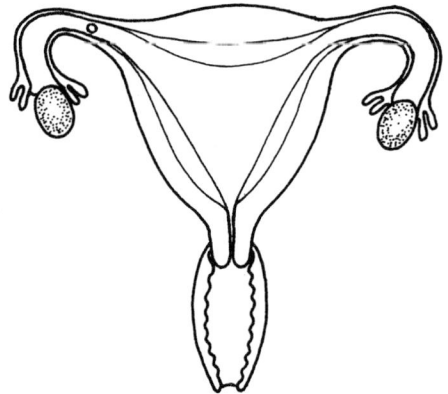

2 Egg travels down fallopian tube

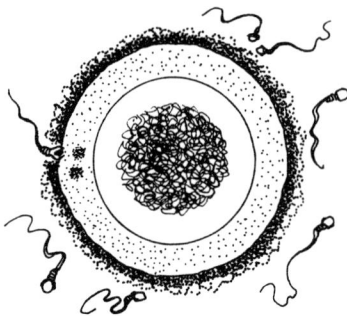

3 Egg is fertilized by sperm

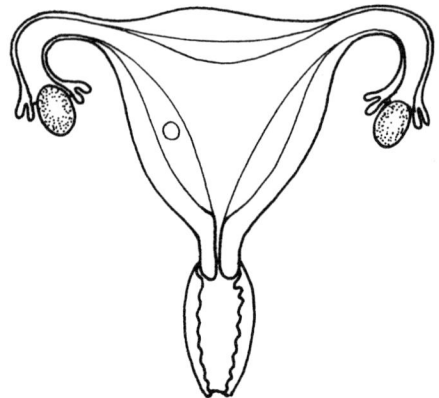

4 Fertilized egg implants in womb

is fertilized, it then has to be able to travel along the fallopian tube to the uterus. A second hormone, progesterone, must be released from the ovary as the egg starts to travel through the fallopian tube, to prepare the endometrium (lining of the womb) for possible implantation by a fertilized egg. The lining should become thick and spongy in order to nourish the newly fertilized egg. Finally, the egg must then implant in the endometrium, where it grows first into an embryo and then into a foetus.

It may be that you have no reason to think that all of these things are not happening perfectly normally. On the other hand, if you are having difficulty in conceiving you need to look at your own circumstances and whether there is anything in your medical history which might interfere with this usual course of events and prevent you from getting pregnant. If you are having very heavy periods or if you have had an infection in the uterus or fallopian tubes at some time, you may want medical assurance that there is no interference with ovulation (egg production) or blockage in the tubes. While you may have read that it is usual to wait for several months before getting help with a fertility problem, you should feel perfectly free to consult your doctor at any time you think there are symptoms which could prevent you from getting pregnant.

The same holds true for your partner. If he has a history of illness which you fear may prevent you getting pregnant, there is no reason to delay asking for medical help. Your medical adviser may want to check out any past infection or illness such as mumps, which can affect a man's testicles. Or if you have difficulty with intercourse, don't wait to 'see what happens'. This will simply make you both tense and anxious.

As well as the conditions being right for conception to occur, you have to remember that there are only a few days each month when you are very fertile and when intercourse has a good chance of leading to pregnancy. The fertile time is some time in the middle of the cycle, around ovulation. But there are ways of pinpointing precisely when ovulation is likely to happen and, using that information, ensuring that you have intercourse during that period. It is interesting to note that there are a number of cases of couples, having difficulty getting pregnant, who have discovered that they were simply not having sex at the right time.

How to get pregnant

It may come as a surprise to many people who have always thought in terms of avoiding pregnancy to realize that there is only a very limited period each month in which the woman is fertile and open to conception. The egg released by the ovary each month is swept into the fallopian tube and it is here that fertilization takes place. It is now thought that the egg can only be fertilized for a very brief period, perhaps even less than 24 hours; the man's sperm can, however, live in the woman's womb and tubes for two or three days. Ideally, then, the sperm should be waiting for the egg to arrive. All this means that there are only two or three days in the month when fertilization can actually occur.

It is possible to predict the moment of ovulation and thus maximize, in theory, the chance of conception occurring. This can be done by the same methods which are used to predict the fertile time in the month for people who wish to avoid pregnancy – the 'rhythm method' of contraception (or natural family planning). The woman's basal body temperature drops slightly just before ovulation and then rises to a higher level for the rest of the menstrual cycle, and this can be measured using an accurate thermometer. The woman has to take her temperature every day immediately on waking, before she gets up or has anything to eat or drink, to make sure that the reading is an accurate one. After three months, if she has a regular cycle, she should be able to predict when ovulation will occur.

The problem with taking readings is that by the time the woman's temperature shows the telltale drop and rise, it is too late for fertilization to occur. The sperm should already be waiting in the tubes for the newly-released egg. So a couple should make love before the chart shows ovulation has occurred, which of course involves guesswork unless you use some other indicator too (see below). By concentrating too much on the right time to make love, a couple can become anxious and inhibited about sex and this might work against conception.

Indeed, some doctors have found that incorrect use of temperature charts may have been the reason why a couple have not conceived. Unless there is evidence of infertility, it is probably best to avoid the use of temperature charts, especially, as it can cause problems in a relationship:

> The temperature charts started to dominate our sex life, and we had endless rows because John was too tired just on the night when I had worked out we had the best chance, or had to go away on business just at the most fertile time in my cycle.

> We just seemed to lose all spontaneity and sex became a mechanical process. It seemed to have less and less to do with how we were feeling. In the end we just threw the thermometer away and had sex when we felt like it.

Women can also recognize when they are fertile by noting the change in the quality of their cervical mucus, which is produced throughout the cycle. When a woman is fertile, the mucus becomes thin, slippery, transparent and more copious, to aid the passage of sperm from the vagina and into the womb – at other times of the month the mucus is normally fairly sticky and forms an effective plug to the entrance of the womb. The presence of sperm in the vagina or any kind of vaginal infection will also make feeling the changes in cervical mucus much more difficult, or even impossible. However, this is still a much better way of telling when you are fertile than temperature charts, although it does mean that you have to test for and be aware of the changes over several days.

There are various chemical tests being developed which will help women tell when they are fertile; dipsticks which change colour when dipped into a woman's urine and more scientific ways of assessing the cervical mucus, but none of these are yet commercially available.

Time to get help?

If you have been trying for some time to get pregnant but with no success, you may have reached the point where you know you are having difficulty and you may be asking yourself, 'Am I infertile?' You may feel that the time has come to do something which may help you find out if there is a serious problem preventing you from getting pregnant.

Most couples who experience this kind of dawning realization that they might not have the child that they are hoping for, go through a period of shock, anxiety and feelings of failure. It can be particularly devastating for a woman who has pursued a career if she feels guilty for having done so at the cost of having a family. One woman in her middle thirties, who had a successful career behind her, described how she felt: 'It was as if it was a punishment – that I was somehow having to pay for all those years when my friends had been submerged in babies and I was out in a man's world.'

A past event may be resurrected and blamed as the cause of the infertility, bringing its own feelings of guilt. One young woman described how she re-lived the memory of an abortion she had had ten years previously:

I hadn't thought about it until I was trying to have a baby. Suddenly it all came back and I was convinced that something must have gone wrong when I had the abortion.

I was angry at myself for post-poning it, but the worst bit was that I had had an abortion when I was twenty and this was one of the things I felt very sad about – that this could have been the cause. Abortions were really difficult to get and I had had it privately. I was sure that some of the scarring was from that. I felt guilty about having abused my body to that extent. But remembering why I had done it, there was no way I could have done anything else. So it was all bringing all that old stuff back.

The fact is that most people do plan their lives around having children at some stage and it does come as a great blow to couples of any age if they think they may be infertile. A woman in her thirties may be tempted to put her infertility down to some problem she has which is related to her age and leave it at that. In fact, the evidence shows that infertility problems are just as likely to be the result of the man being infertile. The assumption is often made that the problem is the woman's, but this is far from the reality. The medical evidence suggests that in one third of infertility cases the problem lies with the man, a third with the woman and in the rest the problem is likely to be both the man and the woman. In about 10 per cent of couples no cause can be found. Added to this, while the question of a woman's age does make some difference to her fertility, it is not so marked as to assume that investigation and treatment are not worth while. However, since infertility assessments and treatments can last some time, hospitals may become increasingly reluctant to perform complicated surgery or therapy as a woman becomes older.

We went to the infertility clinic and had all sorts of tests. They said, 'You're above the age (I was 39) where we do ops and things – we just do the basic tests. All the basic tests showed that I probably had blocked tubes. So they said there was nothing they could do, and I just had the last interview with the doctor who said that they were not prepared to do any more and that, 'you won't get pregnant.' One month later I was.

Getting medical help

Infertility is not uncommon at any age, but women who have waited until their thirties may feel a sense of urgency about getting medical advice and help. Medical investigations can diagnose the causes of infertility and effective treatment is possible. While it cannot be claimed that every couple can be helped, many infertile couples do eventually become parents.

Some women who have been attending their family-planning clinic often find that their first step for seeking help is to raise the matter with a doctor there. But apart from advice, family-planning clinics can do little other than refer you either to your own doctor or to a special fertility clinic.

If you do go to your family doctor, it is probably a good idea to make an appointment for both you and your partner, since the GP will want to see you both at some time. Starting on a series of investigations about your fertility is daunting: you will have to be prepared to answer a whole lot of very personal questions about your sex life as well as go through a number of examinations. Preparing yourself for such 'intrusions' may not necessarily make them any less difficult, but it may help you to ask the right questions and find it easier to talk about personal matters.

Your doctor will want a complete medical history of both you and your partner and will ask you detailed questions about your sex life, how often you have intercourse and whether you have any pain or discomfort at the time of intercourse. You will probably also be given a general examination to check that your health is satisfactory as well as a pelvic examination which will identify any immediate problems such as a discharge. Your partner will also be examined for any physical problems. He may be advised about overweight, drinking and smoking habits, as these have been shown to have a marked effect on fertility.

Many doctors believe that stress, anxiety and over-tiredness are possible causes of infertility and you may be given advice that seems trivial in view of your perception of the problem as a serious one. Your GP may offer advice about ovulation and the best time for intercourse. You may also be asked to keep a temperature chart as described earlier.

After these initial investigations, your doctor may refer you to a specialist clinic that deals with fertility problems.

The causes of infertility

Infertility in women

Inevitably women who fail to conceive quickly after coming off the pill or after using an IUD (intra-uterine device) begin to worry that long-term use of contraception itself is the cause of their failure to conceive. Similarly, women who have had an induced abortion in the past may think that this has affected their fertility.

The evidence is that for the vast majority, contraception does not affect a woman's fertility. However, there has been concern in recent years that the IUD is linked to the increased risk of a woman contracting pelvic inflammatory disease. This is an infection of the fallopian tubes which can lead to infertility if left untreated, and doctors have been increasingly reluctant to fit an IUD in a woman who has not had children.

The contraceptive pill has not been shown to cause infertility, although a woman coming off the pill may find that it takes some time for her periods to return to normal. Some women go for several months without having a period at all before their normal monthly cycle is re-established. But in almost all cases a woman's fertility will return to what it was before taking the pill within a maximum of two years and usually sooner than this.

If there is a risk of abortion causing infertility, it is associated with the risk of an infection at the time of the operation. The chance of infection is about 5 per cent. In some cases an infection may lead to infertility, but the risk of this occurring is the same as the risk of infection during a spontaneous abortion or miscarriage or during childbirth. A recent study shows that early abortion holds no risk for the next pregnancy or future conception.

Smoking may have a small but significant effect on fertility. A recent large study on the effect of age, cigarette smoking and other factors showed that five years after stopping contraception only one in 20 women who were non-smokers had failed to have a child, compared with one in ten who smoked twenty or more cigarettes a day.

One of the major causes of infertility in women is hormone deficiencies or imbalances. These can interfere with the development of the egg in the ovaries or their release. Many women who do not ovulate, or do so irregularly, may already be aware of infrequent or light periods, although some women who do not ovulate regularly do bleed and can have quite heavy periods.

Damage to the fallopian tubes or structural abnormalities may cause a blockage which prevents the sperm from reaching the eggs or prevents the fertilized egg from passing along the fallopian tube to the uterus. Damage to fallopian tubes can be caused by infections which can occur without the woman ever knowing. The most common infection is pelvic inflammatory disease (PID). After the infection has cleared up there may be scarring of the tissue. Sexually transmitted diseases such as chlamydia and gonorrhoea can also cause blocked tubes if not treated promptly. Other causes of damage to the tubes include previous abdominal surgery for such things as appendicitis or ovarian cysts. One leading infertility specialist has criticized surgeons for failing to take sufficient care when performing abdominal surgery to avoid such damage.

Scar tissue may fix the tubes, or the ovaries, or the womb in unnatural positions and make conception impossible. Even if the tubes are not completely blocked, their delicate structure may be damaged in such a way that they are unable to fulfil the function of carrying egg, or sperm, or the fertilized egg to the womb.

Endometriosis is a condition which can result in infertility. It is caused by patches of the lining of the womb (the endometrium) being deposited outside the uterus. This tissue sometimes grows on the ovaries and may form cysts. If the ends of the fallopian tubes are blocked, or if there are adhesions which prevent the tube from being close enough to the ovary, the egg will be unable to enter the fallopian tubes.

There are other causes of infertility, such as abnormalities of the shape of the uterus, which may prevent an egg from implanting and developing. In some cases, women may be born with such abnormalities or they can be the result of fibroids – benign (non-cancerous) lumps which sometimes grow in the uterus and which can prevent conception or interfere with pregnancy, causing a miscarriage.

One form of infertility is secondary or 'second child' infertility, where a woman cannot have another child after one successful pregnancy. Often this may be caused by damage to the womb or tubes during or after childbirth, and can be no less distressing to the woman than primary infertility:

> At least we have Matthew if we don't have another. It's funny – the feelings about wanting a second child are no less intense than feelings about wanting to conceive a first child. I think that would be hard for a childless couple to understand – they would probably give anything to have just one child. But when it comes time to think about another, you want that second child every bit as you wanted the first child.

Other women find that having one child, their lives are not so empty as if they had none:

> I didn't join the NAC (National Association for the Childless). I had a

child and I felt that although it was just as important to me as though I hadn't had one, I felt that other people wouldn't appreciate that, that they would turn round and say, 'Well, what are you talking about? You haven't had the experience. If we had one we would be happy.' So I felt different and so much of my life was involved with mothers with young children. My life was quite full – it wasn't a great chasm or anything.

Infertility in men

Although it is generally the case that in one third of all infertility cases, the problem lies with the man, the causes of infertility in men are less well understood. However, it is known that male infertility has nothing whatsoever to do with a man's virility.

The male reproductive system, like the woman's, is controlled by hormones produced by the body. Testosterone, which is produced in the testes, is responsible for the development of male characteristics – hair growth, deep voice, muscular shape and development, as well as sperm production. Sperm are produced in very large quantities all of the time inside the testes. They then pass into the epididymis where they remain until they become motile (capable of swimming or moving). From there they pass along the tube called the vas deferens where they combine with other secretions (seminal fluid) produced by the glands at the top of the vas deferens before being ejaculated during sexual intercourse. Although the process is a continuous one, it takes something like

three months for sperm to be produced. Unlike a woman, who produces one or possibly two eggs each month, the man produces millions of sperm, and although only one is necessary to fertilize an egg, he is able to ejaculate something like three hundred million sperm at any one time.

Male reproductive organs

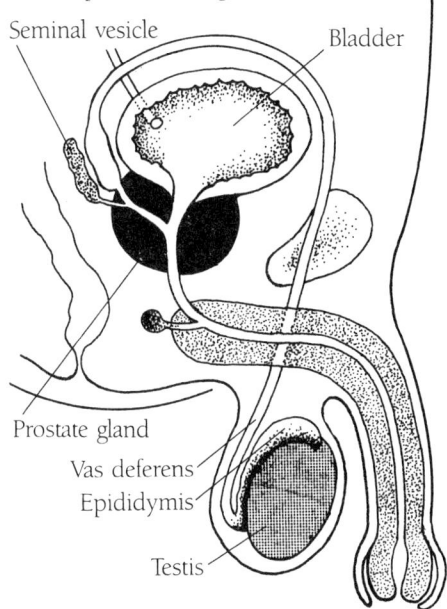

But factors other than simple quantity of sperm are important. While all men produce a large number of sperm which are abnormal in some way or not motile, there may be difficulty in the woman conceiving if a man does not produce a sufficient number of normally formed or normally motile sperm or an adequate amount of seminal fluid.

The testes themselves are contained in a bag of skin known as the scrotum, which hangs outside the body. This allows them to maintain a temperature slightly lower than the rest of the body, which is necessary for sperm production. One of the simplest, but not obvious, causes of male infertility is a rise in temperature of the testes which leads to a drop in sperm production. Tight-fitting underwear, trousers or jeans can be the cause of a temperature rise. So, too, can doing certain kinds of jobs in very hot conditions. These things may produce only temporary fertility problems which are easily rectified. But there are other risks of damage to the testicles which men run, through accident or injury. Congenital conditions, illnesses such as mumps leading to inflammation of the testicles (orchitis) can lead to low sperm production. Undescended testicles in childhood can be a further cause of infertility. Infections including sexually transmitted diseases, which are not treated promptly can lead to blocked ducts and tubes. A few men are also known to produce antibodies which kill off their own sperm especially after vasectomy reversal or an operation to open up blocked tubes.

Varicocele is probably the commonest single cause of male infertility, as between 30 and 40 per cent of infertile men have this varicose vein of the testicle. No one is quite sure how it affects fertility, but in 10 per cent of men with varicocele infertility is the result. One theory is that the larger quantity of blood in the vein overheats the testicle and affects sperm production.

Infertility - a joint problem

Some infertility problems are caused by the inability of the sperm to survive in the woman's body. For conception to occur, the sperm have to be able to swim through the woman's cervical mucus. The woman's vagina is in fact a hostile environment for the man's sperm. It is usually more acid than sperm like, but they are normally protected from this by the alkalinity of the seminal fluid. Sometimes the woman's vagina can be too acid for the sperm to survive well in it - either because of a minor infection or because of the woman's own body chemistry.

The cervix - the opening to the uterus - is protected from infections by the cervical mucus which in its usual form is thick and tacky. Normally the passage of the sperm is made easier around the time of ovulation, the cervical mucus becoming thinner, more copious and more fluid. The changes in the consistency of the cervical mucus are controlled by the production in the body of the hormones oestrogen and progesterone. Just before ovulation the oestrogen level reaches a peak. After ovulation the level of progesterone rises again and the mucus returns to its thicker, tackier consistency.

Infertility can also be caused by a woman producing antibodies to her partner's sperm. The body normally produces antibodies to protect itself from infections. But it is thought that the body sometimes reacts in this way to certain harmless substances and produces antibodies. If this happens, then the antibodies effectively kill off the sperm:

In fact what I was tested for in the end was sperm antibodies. Once they knew that, I got treatment and I was pregnant the first month. They treated it with cortisone – it was just one month of very mild cortisone tablets and I was pregnant. At that stage it was a case of 'You've got this far, you might as well try it,' but without any real hopes.

Infertility tests

At the infertility clinic both partners will be asked again for details of their previous illnesses, operations and sex life. Although this may be embarrassing, it is necessary for accurate diagnosis and all the information is completely confidential. (It might be important to know that a man had got a woman pregnant or a woman had had an abortion, although neither partner might wish the other to know this.) A routine physical examination will be done to find out about your partner's and your own state of health, including taking a urine sample, checking blood pressure and weight.

A variety of techniques have been developed for finding out how the male and female reproductive systems are working and, at a later stage, more detailed investigation may follow.

One of the first tests of infertility is to find out whether the woman is ovulating, so you may be asked to keep temperature charts. But because this is not a precise measure, you will probably also be given further tests to measure the level of hormones which control ovulation. A blood progesterone test, which is a simple and painless way of measuring the amount of progesterone, may be done. This measures the level of progesterone when it reaches its peak at about day 24 in a 28-day cycle. If the level of progesterone is high, it is a good indication that you have ovulated.

The post-coital test is another simple procedure which may help pinpoint why you are not conceiving. You will be asked to make an appointment for a time of the month when you are ovulating. You will be asked to have sexual intercourse on the previous night or the morning of your appointment before you go to the clinic for the test. At the clinic the doctor will take a sample of the cervical mucus from the neck of the womb, and by examining this he will be able to tell a number of things. The quality of the mucus will indicate whether you are ovulating (producing eggs). By examining the mucus under a microscope, he will be able to tell if your partner is producing normal sperm, how many there are and whether there are antibodies against sperm. If post-coital tests are repeatedly not very good, the next step may be to test the semen and the mucus for antibodies to sperm which may interfere with the sperm's normal motility.

Another, more complicated, procedure for looking at the woman's hormone levels is to take a small sample of the lining of the uterus for examination. This minor surgical procedure (similar to a 'D and C') is called an endometrial biopsy. The purpose is to inspect the quality of ovulation and receptiveness of the uterus to egg implantation. If all these test show that you are ovulating normally, you may then go through a series of tests to find out whether all the reproductive organs are functioning.

You may have an X-ray of the uterus and fallopian tubes taken by injecting a dye through the cervix and into the uterus. The dye passes through the uterus, along the fallopian tubes and into the pelvic cavity. The procedure is called a hysterosalpingram, and the X-ray shows what happens to the dye as it passes through. It will show any abnormality of the uterus and whether the tubes are clear. If one or both tubes are blocked, the movement of the dye is obstructed.

One technique which is used to detect blocked or damaged tubes is laparoscopy. This has to be done under general anaesthetic. A small incision is made in the navel and a laporoscope, which is a telescope-like instrument, is used to examine the ovaries, the uterus and the fallopian tubes.

The quality of the man's semen will also be tested as a first step to see whether the sperm are healthy, numerous and sufficiently motile. (Very often this is the only test which the man will undergo, unlike the woman who may be required to go on attending the clinic over a long period of time.) The man will be asked to produce a specimen of his semen and he will be asked to do this by masturbating into a container provided by the clinic. The sample has then to be delivered to the laboratory where it is examined soon after it is produced. If the sperm count and test indicate that his semen is of good quality, then he may not be involved in any further examinations. If, on the other hand, the sperm count is low or the sperm are not vigorous, further tests may follow. The sperm may also be examined, by means of a post-coital test, to see how they survive inside the woman's body. This test may give some idea about why the sperm are not functioning properly.

In some cases the man may have a scrototomy. This is an operation carried out under general anaesthetic to open up the scrotum and see whether there are any abnormalities or obstructions.

Treatments for infertility in women

There are many forms of treatment for infertility and what may be appropriate for one couple may not work for another. However, many couples can be helped to achieve a pregnancy. Some treatments, such as IVF (in vitro fertilization) or GIFT (gamete intra-fallopian transfer) are now available giving various rates of success.

For women who have problems ovulating, drug treatment through the use of the so-called 'fertility drugs' offers a good chance of boosting hormone production and starting ovulation again. The main drawback of one of these drugs (Pergonal) is the risk of a multiple pregnancy. In the majority of cases the risk is of twins, but occasionally triplets (or more) are born to women who take this drug and these cases are often reported in the press.

The most widely used fertility drug is clomiphene (brand name Clomid) which seems to induce ovulation in about 80 per cent of women treated, though not all of these achieve pregnancy. The drug is usually given for five days in the early part of a woman's cycle to induce ovulation. It has been in use for many years and seems very safe though a few women have unpleasant side-effects: 'I had weird symptoms while taking the drug and they said it was all in my head. Later I asked a gynaecologist friend what were the side-effects of this drug and he listed all the things I had been feeling!'

Pergonal, the brand name for the naturally occurring human menopausal gonadotrophin, a hormone produced by menopausal women, will induce about 90 per cent of women to ovulate. About 20–30 per cent of pregnancies resulting from this drug will be twins or more, and it can have unpleasant side-effects. Occasionally women have to be hospitalized with over-stimulated ovaries.

Another drug which can help some women who do not ovulate with either of these drugs is bromocriptine. This seems to work in women who, for some reason, have a high level of a hormone called prolactin in their blood – this hormone is normally produced when women are breast-feeding.

It is possible to correct tubal damage by surgery, although the success rates vary. Tubal surgery is a difficult and delicate operation and is only per-formed by a small number of surgeons. Fallopian tubes can be repaired and scar tissue and fibroids removed by delicate operations using techniques involving microsurgery. But the outcome of surgery depends on how much damage there is. Little can be done, for example, if the lining of the tubes or the delicate fimbriae at the ends of the tubes are damaged.

In recent years, the progress which medical science has made in developing in vitro fertilization (IVF or the 'test tube baby' technique, as it has been known) or GIFT has offered new hope for women unable to conceive because of blocked or damaged tubes. As long as a woman's ovaries are functioning normally and she has a healthy uterus, this technique offers a way of bypassing blocked tubes. It involves removing a number of eggs from the woman's ovaries at a time of the month when they are mature and ready to be released. The eggs and the man's sperm are brought together in a culture dish in the lab – the reason why the technique is known as the 'test tube baby' treatment. This is then transferred to an incubator for twenty-four hours. If the eggs are of good quality and the sperm normal, fertilization will most likely take place. One or more fertilized eggs are then inserted into the womb – the more eggs there are the better the chance of conception as the eggs seem to stimulate one another's growth, but the greater the risk of a multiple pregnancy.

With this treatment, more eggs are fertilized than may be needed. This may mean that the frozen eggs are available for further treatment if the first attempt is unsuccessful or if the pregnancy is not maintained. But the question which has arisen recently is that of what happens to them if they are not used in this way? One possibility, which offers hope to women with little prospect of having a baby at the moment, is that they could be made available and donated to women whose fertility problems are caused by their inability to produce eggs, but who may be able to carry a pregnancy and give birth. Another recent development is GIFT – gamete intra-fallopian transfer. This technique involves the transfer of egg and sperm back into the fallopian tubes where it is hoped fertilization will take place. This avoids some of the problems of IVF.

Needless to say, there is much concern and controversy about the ethical issues involved in IVF. Similarly, the question of surrogate mothering has recently raised many complex questions. Surrogate motherhood is seen by some as offering a solution where the woman is the infertile partner. Through artificial insemination, the husband or partner fertilizes a woman who is prepared to carry the child but who hands it over at birth to the father and his wife. The legal, ethical and moral questions are complex – the law is not clear about such contracts and cannot resolve any difficulties which may arise if there are problems with the pregnancy itself or if the child is born handicapped. There has also been concern over the question of payments and the growth of agencies set up to make contractual arrangements of this kind. The whole question of exploitation and profiting from such situations is viewed by many as being undesirable.

Treatments for infertility in men

If the cause of infertility lies with the man, and since less is known about male infertility, the chances of successful treatment are not as great as when the problem lies with the woman.

It has been thought that hormonal problems similar to those which prevent ovulation in women might be the cause of low sperm counts in men. As a result, a variety of drugs used successfully on women – clomiphene, HMG and HCG– have been tried on men but with no real evidence of success. Another therapy which was tried is testosterone rebound, where doses of testosterone were given to depress sperm production, and its withdrawal was supposed to stimulate new sperm production to greater levels than before treatment. Results of this treatment are no more encouraging. They may work in some cases, but there appears to be no clear explanation as to why they work. Nevertheless many men will feel that any treatment is worth trying if it offers some hope, however small, of success.

There are techniques of making sure that the sperm have the best possible chance of fertilizing an egg – if the problem is that of a low sperm count. The man's own semen can be artificially introduced into the woman's vagina, depositing it high in the vagina or at the entrance to the cervix. An added measure is to concentrate the sperm from several ejaculations or use the 'split ejaculate' technique where the woman is fertilized with only the first part of the semen. This contains 80 per cent of the sperm and is more alkaline, which may help sperm survival.

Surgery to overcome blockages in the epididymis or vas deferens is sometimes performed but, again, the success rates are low. However, if the infertility is thought to be caused by a varicocele (a varicose vein at the top of the testis which accounts for about 30 per cent of male infertility), there is a good chance of cure. A varicocele may not be obvious and may require careful examination before it is detected. Simple surgery to tie off the affected vein usually brings about a marked increase in sperm production, although it will take from three to six months to ascertain the results. The quality and number of sperm improves in about 80 per cent of men treated, but only about half of these will succeed in starting a pregnancy – the higher the sperm count before the operation, the greater the chances of success afterwards.

If a man is completely sterile, artificial insemination by donor is a possible solution which a couple may wish to consider. This is now a well-established technique, with relatively high success rates. More than 50 per cent of women who are treated in this way conceive. Semen is provided by an anonymous donor and is introduced artificially into the woman's vagina during the fertile period of her cycle.

The semen is very carefully tested for quality and to ensure that it is free of any virus, such as the acquired immune deficiency syndrome (AIDS) virus. In selecting sperm, every effort is made to match the characteristics of the donor with those of the partner – hair and eye colour, height and blood group – so that the child might bear a similar resemblance to the man who will bring it up as his own. Donors are also carefully screened to make sure that there are no genetic problems which might affect a child, and that they are young, intelligent, healthy and psychologically well balanced.

However, although artificial insemination technology is now relatively simple, there are considerable drawbacks in having a baby this way. In the first place, the procedure is not readily available on the NHS and many couples seek the help of the private clinics rather than join the long waiting lists. There is also considerable confusion surrounding the legal status, rights and claims of the child and the question of who is the legal father. Linked to the legal questions are the ethical concerns which many people have about artificial insemination. These concerns have not yet been openly discussed and for the most part it is an issue which has been shrouded in secrecy. All of this means that the implications for a couple considering AID are very complex and they may need a great deal of time and counselling to be sure that AID parenthood is what they want. Most important of all are the social and emotional problems. It is very difficult for some men to father a child who is not his biological child, and it may take some time for him to be sure that he is going to be able to accept the child as his and to father him in a way that he would if he were his own.

It is also very stressful for a woman to go through pregnancy carrying a child without knowing who the biological father is. Further, there is the question of the child's right to know about his or her origins; adopted people now have the right to know about their natural parents, and it is felt that more openness about AID would benefit all concerned. Nevertheless, there are many couples who have worked through all the difficulties associated with AID and who in the end have happily had a baby this way.

Problems with infertility investigations

The whole process of infertility investigations can be very harrowing. The very nature of the tests themselves can create anxiety and stress. Waiting will be an inevitable part of the process, since many of the tests have to be done at certain times of the month.

> It was all a question of trial and error. I had one kind of test and then went back. It was a difficult time. The longer it went on the more obsessive you got about it. Examining everything in detail makes you obsessive.

Appointments not only have to be made at different times in the menstrual cycle; some may have to be repeated. Some of the tests may prevent a couple from having intercourse at the fertile time of the month, which further delays possible conception, so they are often spaced out for this reason. Many couples in fact conceive while investigations are going on and some doctors like to give time for this to occur and prevent unnecessary invasive operations:

> I felt rather stupid. I was booked for a post-coital test the following month, but when my period didn't start I didn't go. I went back to see the consultant and he asked me angrily why I hadn't gone, but he was delighted when I gave the reason.

The whole process can be drawn out over one, two or even more years. It is the determination to have a baby which gives women the incentive to carry on and to go back repeatedly to the clinic:

> You need an incredible commitment to go through it all. There was one point when I was having blood tests and cervical mucus tests and everything, when I had to be at the hospital every morning for weeks on end at eight-thirty. So that needs a commitment when you are really busy. Trailing backwards and forwards and making arrangements for the child – for Tom to be late at work. Other people were travelling to hospital to be there at eight-thirty in the morning. It weeded out the people, by virtue of that, that really wanted a child.

With so many different forms of

investigations and tests, treatment will vary according to the individual's particular problem. No two cases are the same. But anyone who is not entirely happy with their treatment or who feels that they would like a second opinion can ask for this. For one woman, who had a good idea what was wrong with her, this turned out to be a wise move:

> I read books on infertility and I had a friend who went to the same clinic but saw a different doctor. He gave her every conceivable test and was going to the ends of the earth to help her. Her case was no different, she had one child the same age as mine. It was just the different doctor. She had got the brush-off from the same doctor as me. Eventually I diagnosed myself, having discovered that I had endometriosis, and I went to the GP and told him. I would have thought that they would have checked that out but they hadn't. If I hadn't agitated and said, 'Look I've got this'. . . . I was put on a course of drugs. They certainly didn't guarantee anything would happen as a result, but as it happened I did get pregnant. So I was treated for endometriosis after four years of failed infertility treatment.

The stress involved in trying to have a child, sometimes hoping against hope, does put unbearable pressure on relationships and there may come a time where the stress does become too much and has to be relieved in some way. Some couples reach a point themselves when they begin to look at the issue in a different light:

But there had to be a point in my mind where I had to accept rather than bash my head against a closed door and deal with how we were going to cope with not having children. I think I had set myself a target that I would at least have a laparoscopy to see what it was, and I wouldn't have gone beyond a simple operation – the test-tube thing – although a friend of mine was going through that and I kept saying, 'You're crazy.' But for me it was more important to look at why I was so desperate and how I was going to cope and what to do instead. Should we adopt? Or throw ourselves into being a good uncle and aunt?

In many cases it is other people who may help a couple, trying hard to have a baby, to see things differently:

> The GP said something interesting: 'Just accept the fact that you haven't got what you wanted anyway.' So that took a bit of pressure off us. That was quite helpful – 'Just take what you get,' he said.
>
> I always wanted them to find something wrong rather than say, 'There's nothing wrong.' If they found something I would know one way or the other. It was that sort of sense of not knowing. But the depression about it all was relieved by what the doctor said – but we still wanted another baby. It was almost as if I was wasting time. I was biding time during that time and not really getting on with life. If I had known that I was only going to have James, I would

have accepted that much more quickly and been happy about only having one child. But I don't regret that time now because I had Mark in the end, but I think I would have regretted if it I hadn't had Mark.

Because it is usually the woman who has to go through the months of investigations, finding moral support does help. Most women want the support of their partner even though he may not be required for the clinic appointment. You may also find that one of the best ways of relieving the stress for both you and your partner is by getting together with other people in a similar situation through self-help organizations. The National Association for the Childless puts people at different stages of infertility investigation in touch with one another. Many of their members find that just discussing their experiences and apprehensions enables them to cope with the distressing aspects of infertility investigations, and sharing some of the embarrassing side often allows them to treat some of these tests in a light-hearted and even humorous way.

You may wish to find out for yourself what facilities exist in your area. There are a number of agencies which can provide this information. The National Association for the Childless keeps a register of infertility clinics, as does the Family Planning Association and your community health council or local health council.

If you are referred to a specialist clinic for investigations and treatment, you may want to find out details of how quickly you are likely to be seen. The services vary around the country and some of them do have enormously long waiting lists. Time may be of the essence as far as you are concerned and you may wish to find out what services are available privately. However, you may be lucky and find yourself in a part of the country where there is considerable research interest in this area and you may have the advantage of all the new technology.

Miscarriage

There are many women who have a problem at some time of carrying a pregnancy to full term and lose the baby early in the pregnancy. The loss of a baby before 28 weeks of pregnancy is referred to as a spontaneous abortion in medical terms, but most women use the term miscarriage.

It is important to remember that miscarriage is a very common occurrence. Between one in five and one in seven women who know that they are pregnant will have a miscarriage, and in most cases – about 85 per cent – it happens very early in the pregnancy, usually before the twelfth week is over. Yet, that does not alter the fact that losing a baby at whatever stage is very distressing.

The first thing you are likely to notice if you have a miscarriage is bleeding. It may start with no warning at all. The blood loss may be slight to begin with or there may be a heavy flow. You may also experience cramp-like pains, which can be quite severe, in the lower part of your back as the uterus begins to contract. If there is no pain and only a small blood loss and if the placenta remains attached to the wall of the uterus, the miscarriage may be only a threatened miscarriage and the pregnancy may continue, although you may have to rest in bed or in hospital.

I was very worried while I was pregnant. I started bleeding and was absolutely frantic. I stayed in bed convinced that this was a punishment from the gods. Then I discovered that it – bleeding – is not uncommon. I was lucky; I stayed in bed for a week and everything was fine. After that I had a perfectly normal pregnancy and the baby was fine – nothing wrong at all.

Some miscarriages can happen quite quickly and relatively painlessly while other women experience miscarriages which go on for several days and are very painful:

It happened very suddenly. I was three months pregnant and very happy, looking forward to our first baby. I was feeling a bit tired but we had had an evening out, visiting friends. When we came home I bent down to pick something up from the floor and I realized I was bleeding. I panicked but managed to ring the doctor who told me to go to bed and rest and stay as still as possible. I did, but every time I got up there would be a little bit more bleeding. I stayed in bed for several days but at the end of the week I woke up with very bad pain in my back. I rang the doctor and they took me into hospital. The pain was really bad – I suppose it was like being in labour – and eventually I passed a lot of blood. Then I had a D and C as they said the miscarriage was not complete.

I felt very tired, but worse than that – just so terrible and quite devastated by it.

If you do have bleeding or severe pain or both, you should see your doctor. He may think it advisable to send you to hospital. In cases where miscarriage is incomplete, it is necessary to have a D and C (dilation and curettage) which is a scraping of the womb and is done to ensure that nothing is left behind and to prevent any infection which could affect the woman's future fertility.

Grief and loss

Apart from the physical reaction and feeling very tired after a miscarriage there are the feelings of depression and grief. The sense of loss and bereavement may last for several months or indeed until a successful pregnancy occurs, and for most couples it takes time for the process to be worked through. These genuine feelings of grief need to be acknowledged so that they can be resolved. Support groups such as the Miscarriage Association may provide invaluable help.

Perhaps it is because miscarriage is so common that friends and relatives seldom recognize the significance of the loss to a woman and gloss over it. Very often the advice is to 'go ahead and get pregnant again' and implied in this is the idea that this will somehow automatically relieve the distress and allow the couple to 'forget' about the miscarriage. In fact for many this advice is not helpful and is a denial of the very real feelings of grief. Forgetting or blocking out the grief may only mean that it will surface again at some time in the future, causing more confusion as well as distress:

> I suppose I was overconcerned about not getting pregnant again and the hospital said, 'You'll soon have another one.' I tried very hard to get pregnant and when I did, the first thing I felt was guilt about the baby I had lost. It shouldn't have been like that and if I had got over the loss before trying again I think I would have felt better.

A miscarriage, especially if it occurs later in pregnancy, is a real bereavement. But, added to this, many women find that the depression and loss increases in the months after the miscarriage and can be especially acute at the time when the baby was due to be born: 'It was only when the date when she should have been born had passed that I somehow felt the grief begin to subside and that I could put it behind me and begin to think about having another baby.'

The reaction to a miscarriage may be doubly difficult for an older woman if she feels anxious about the possibility of further miscarriages. There does seem to be a slightly greater chance of a woman miscarrying as she gets older, and first pregnancies are also slightly more likely to end in miscarriage. But the fact is that most women, whatever their age, who have one miscarriage will never have another one.

The causes of miscarriage

It is difficult to pinpoint the precise cause of a miscarriage. In about 50 per cent of cases there is something wrong with the foetus and it is thought that the body's rejection of the malformed foetus is nature's way of dealing with the mistake. A chromosomal abnormality such as Down's Syndrome is the most common problem, or the foetus may be damaged in some way which would result in a defect. However, this does not mean that a couple will never be able to have children; some foetuses will still be able to develop normally.

Women who miscarry may hear the term 'blighted egg' or 'blighted ovum' used to explain what went wrong. This means that either the egg or the sperm, which fertilized the egg, was abnormal, so that the fertilized egg failed to develop in the normal way. This will usually result in an early miscarriage.

Women who suffer from certain illnesses, such as heart or kidney disease, or diabetes, may have difficulty in carrying a baby to full term. In most of these cases the condition is known in advance and the woman will be given regular check-ups in the early part of her pregnancy. Smoking and excessive drinking are also thought to make miscarriage slightly more likely.

Another reason for miscarriage may be hormonal problems. Doctors think that a decrease in the levels of the hormone progesterone, which is necessary to sustain a pregnancy, is linked with miscarriage. Some women may have a deficiency of progesterone which is not sufficiently severe to prevent a pregnancy but just severe enough to allow a miscarriage to occur. This can usually be confirmed by taking blood samples to check hormone levels throughout the woman's monthly cycle.

Many miscarriages occur at three months and this is a very delicate time in pregnancy. It is the time when the womb starts to expand as the foetus begins to grow rapidly and when the placenta takes over the task of maintaining hormone levels. If something is not quite right at this point the placenta can become detached from the wall of the uterus, or the hormone levels can fall too low, rejecting the pregnancy.

A miscarriage can also be due to the failure of the womb to expand to accommodate the growing foetus. In a small number of cases a physical abnormality of the uterus, or fibroids, may prevent a foetus from growing beyond a certain stage.

Beyond the first twelve weeks of a pregnancy, miscarriages are usually caused by problems either in the attachment of the placenta to the uterus or an inability of the cervix to cope with the pressure of the foetus as it grows – known as an 'incompetent' cervix. In this case the cervix dilates (opens) and the foetus passes out of the uterus long before it can survive on its own.

Very rarely a woman may suffer repeated miscarriages because her body rejects the baby as a foreign body. This can be because, by chance, her partner and she are genetically similar. A new treatment is now available to overcome this problem.

Preventing a miscarriage

If you have a miscarriage and are anxious about the possibility of a another miscarriage, you will probably want to discuss it with your doctor, although the NHS will seldom investigate the cause of a miscarriage unless you have had three. This is because the vast majority of women who have one or even two miscarriages have a normal pregnancy next time. However, if your age or a previous history of infertility makes conception seem unlikely, you may want to discuss if and how you can prevent another miscarriage. Your doctor may refer you to a specialist for investigations to see if there is any abnormality of the uterus. If there is a suggestion that the cause of miscarriage is genetic, he or she may refer you to a genetic counsellor.

If the miscarriage is caused by the cervix dilating early in the pregnancy, doctors can treat this by putting stitches through the muscles of the cervix, so that it cannot expand. The stitches are then removed a week or two before the baby is due.

Women who have had several miscarriages may be given hormone injections. There are cases where they appear to help some women to carry a baby to full term, but there is concern about the possible side-effects of hormone treatments and opinion is divided about how safe and effective such treatment is. Some doctors are very sceptical about the use of hormone treatments as there is no evidence that they are really helpful; and in some cases there would be no point in trying to prevent miscarriage, since this would simply result in the birth of a handi-capped baby.

Most doctors will give women advice which sounds like good common sense to many and they are happy to go along with it. For example, most will advise bed rest if a miscarriage threatens or as a natural course of action in the early weeks of a pregnancy if a woman has had several previous miscarriages. Al-though there is no evidence that this will necessarily prevent a miscarriage, it will, at the very least, reassure a woman that she is doing nothing to harm the chances of her baby surviving. Similarly, while there is no conclusive evidence about the harmful effects of sexual intercourse in the early weeks of pregnancy, women who have had a previous miscarriage may feel that it makes sense to avoid sexual intercourse, at least until after the stage at which they have previously miscarried.

In general, many women find that the sound advice about 'looking after your-self', and avoiding harmful things like cigarettes and alcohol, are also sensible precautions to take to give themselves the best chance of a healthy pregnancy.

CHAPTER FOUR

Screening for Abnormalities

The development of a human embryo from fertilized egg through to a fully developed baby is a very complex process. There can hardly be a mother who has not worried at some time in her pregnancy whether her baby will be normal, and this may be particularly true for the older mother. Fortunately, there are now a number of screening tests offered to women who are at risk of having an abnormal baby. These tests can be very important in setting the parent's minds at rest or, in cases where an abnormality is shown, in enabling them to decide whether or not to proceed with a pregnancy. However, it is important to remember that not all abnormalities can be detected in pregnancy and that accidents at birth can also lead to handicap. The tests eliminate certain problems but do not guarantee the 'perfect baby'.

How the baby develops

A human embryo is more or less completely formed by the end of the twelfth week of pregnancy. After this time it simply has to grow in size and its organs have to mature to make it capable of life outside the womb. All the major developments take place in the early weeks of pregnancy, which is why it is most important to look after yourself before you even know you are pregnant. The baby's spinal column, for example, is beginning to form in the fifth week of pregnancy. You are likely at this stage to realize that your period is late, but not have had a pregnancy confirmed. In the sixth week arm and leg buds are formed and in the seventh week the beginnings of the fingers and toes are visible and dramatic changes are occurring to the head and face. In the ninth week the nose and mouth take shape and by the eleventh week the genitals are formed, and all the internal organs are functioning.

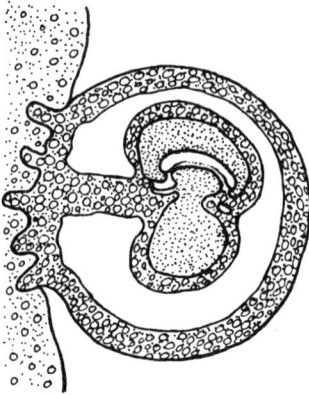

Week 4–5

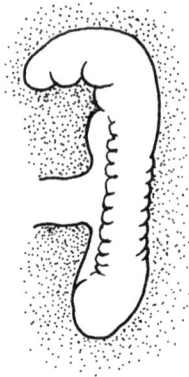

Week 5

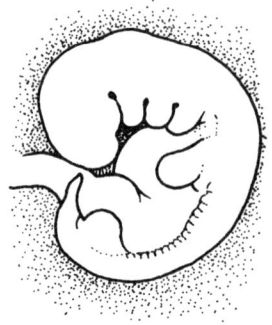

Weeks 6–7

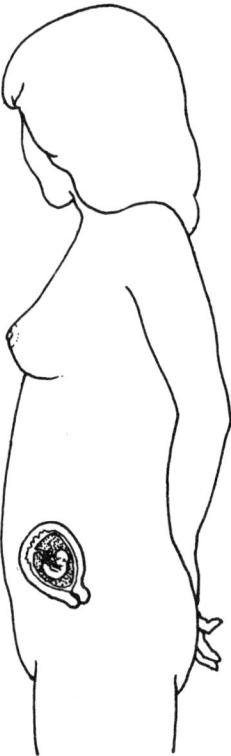

Weeks 8–9

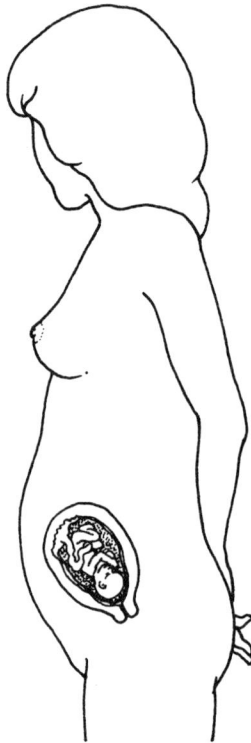

Week 20

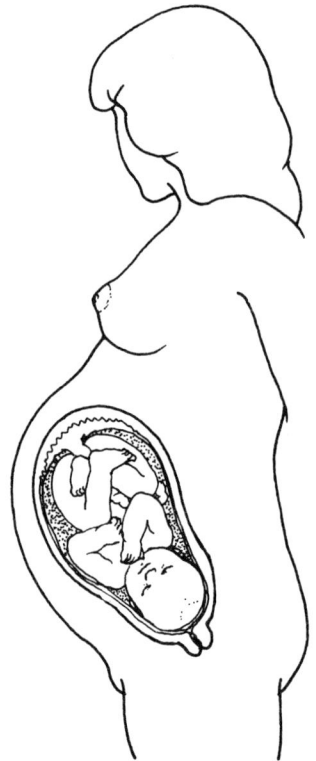

Week 36

How things go wrong

Abnormalities in a baby are usually caused by genetic problems or by an environmental influence, such as poor diet, the use of drugs in early pregnancy or by hazards in the workplace, such as toxic chemicals or radiation. Genetic problems fall into two categories: those which are caused by either or both parents carrying a faulty gene, or those which occur when the sperm or egg are formed and involve an extra chromosome or part of a chromosome being included in the fertilized egg.

Chromosomes are the essential components of every living cell which determine not only how each cell works, but how the whole organism grows, develops, functions and looks. The chromosomes are made up of smaller units called genes, each of which determines a particular characteristic of the organism. Each different animal and plant species has its unique number and size of chromosomes, carrying all the relevant genes. In humans there are 46 chromosomes in 23 pairs. One set is inherited from the mother and one set from the father of each individual.

When the human cells divide to create the sperm or the egg, the pairs of chromosomes are mixed and separated at random so that each egg and each sperm carries a different set of genes, although there will always be one of each pair. This is why every human being is different. One of the pairs of chromosomes determines the baby's sex; these are called the X and Y chromosomes, because of their shape when viewed under the microscope. When sperm are formed, half will carry the Y chromosome which determines maleness, and half the X chromosome. All eggs carry the X chromosome. It is therefore the father who determines the sex of a baby.

Very occasionally the process of division will go wrong and the sperm or egg cell will end up with an extra chromosome, or sometimes an extra part of a chromosome, and when sperm and egg fuse the embryo will be faulty. In most cases these abnormal sperm, eggs or embryos will not be able to survive or, if the embryo does develop, the baby cannot survive long. It is thought that a high proportion – as many as 50 per cent – of miscarriages are caused by the embryo being abnormal.

Sometimes, however, the presence of an extra chromosome does not prevent the baby from developing or living. The most common of these is when there is an extra one of the 21st pair of chromosomes, which causes Down's Syndrome. Other chromosomal abnormalities which are not lethal are when a girl lacks an X chromosome (Turner's Syndrome) or a boy has an extra X or an extra Y chromosome.

Apart from chromosomal abnormalities, other diseases and handicaps are caused by a faulty gene. Literally hundreds of inherited illnesses are now known, although most are extremely rare. Some of these are caused by a dominant gene, others – and these are more common – by a recessive gene.

A dominant gene is one which will always show itself if it is present, while a recessive gene can remain hidden, perhaps for generations. Each individual inherits one gene for each characteristic from each parent. Suppose he inherits one gene for blue eyes and one gene for brown. He clearly cannot have two-colour eyes at the same time, nor is it usual to have one eye of each colour! What happens is that one gene is dominant over the other – brown eyes dominate blue, so the individual has brown eyes. However, he still carries a gene for blue eyes which, if it is paired with another gene for blue eyes in his future partner, can express itself in the next generation.

Two relatively well-known, dominantly inherited diseases are Huntingdon's Chorea, a degenerative nerve disease which does not show up till the third or fourth decade of life, and achondroplasia, a form of dwarfism linked to older fathers. If a person has a dominantly inherited disease, they have a 50 per cent chance of having an affected child.

Recessively inherited diseases are more insidious as they can be carried by large numbers of people without their knowledge. As long as the recessive gene is only paired with normal genes, there is no problem. However, if two people carrying the abnormal gene have children, there is a one-in-four chance of their baby having the disease; and other children are likely to be carriers.

Recessively inherited diseases include cystic fibrosis, Tay Sachs disease, sickle-cell anaemia, and phenylketonuria. Some of these can be treated if diagnosed early (all babies in this country have a tiny pin-prick of blood taken in the first week of life to test for diseases like phenylketonuria). Others can be tested for during pregnancy (see below).

Many genes are carried in the X chromosomes and these cause sex-linked diseases if they are abnormal. If a person is female and has two X chromosomes, the abnormal gene is likely to be masked by a normal gene. If it is paired with a Y chromosome, however, there may be no normal gene to mask it as the Y chromosome is shorter and carries fewer genes. Examples of sex-linked diseases are haemophilia and Duchenne muscular dystrophy.

Some congenital abnormalities are caused not by a simple faulty gene but by a combination of factors. Perhaps several faulty genes are involved, or a combination of a faulty gene with some environmental stimulus such as a drug taken in pregnancy, or a faulty diet. Neural tube defects (anencephaly and spina bifida), cleft palate and hare-lip, and some congenital heart defects are caused in this way. Indeed, there may be a random element, too. There have been recorded cases of identical twins being born where one had a cleft lip and the other did not.

Fortunately, most of these problems are relatively rare. But abnormalities such as Down's Syndrome and spina bifida are more common and more likely to be a cause of concern. On the other hand, these are the abnormalities which can be detected by tests in the early stages of pregnancy.

Down's Syndrome

This is the most common chromosomal abnormality and affects about one in 600 live-born infants in Britain. The most significant problem faced by Down's Syndrome children is that they are mentally handicapped, althought the degree of handicap varies; some can, with help, and stimulation, achieve IQs of about 80, considered to be the dull end of the normal spectrum; many have IQs of less than 50 and are severely mentally handicapped. Down's Syndrome children can also be recognized by their flattened profile, slanted eyes with an extra fold (hence the label Mongol) and stubby fingers. Most grow slowly and are small for their age, and many have additional handicaps – heart defects, eye abnormalities, hearing problems and a tendency to respiratory infections are common. Down's Syndrome babies are characteristically 'floppy' at birth and many have problems with breast-feeding as they may lack strength to feed properly as well as the reflex to suck.

Most women expect to have a normal healthy baby when they go into labour, although a very small number may know that their baby is likely to be born handicapped. When things go wrong and a woman has to face up to this at the time of the birth, the shock and disbelief can be quite devastating:

They told us after the birth that she wasn't normal. I refused to listen. I said, if you're worried about her slanting eyes, my other children had that, they're my husband's eyes. Then they showed me how she didn't have the normal reflexes and how floppy she was and one or two other things, and I had to believe it was true. My husband was also told and he didn't know what to say; we couldn't look at one another. My first feeling for the baby was absolute hate: I hated her for not being normal. I seriously thought of having her adopted. That lasted a day or two.

It may take the parents days, weeks and sometimes even months to accept what has happened and to acknowledge that a baby born with some form of handicap needs just as much love and care as a normal baby:

I wouldn't talk to the other mothers, or the staff, wouldn't see my family, and wouldn't see the baby. Then I thought, she can't be that bad, I'll just go and look at her. She was asleep (the nurses had been feeding her). I just looked and looked at her and she was so tiny, so beautiful, like my other babies had been. I felt a rush of love and when my husband came I was feeding her and crying. I told him, 'we have to keep her, she needs us more than anyone.' He just smiled and smiled and said, 'That's what I've been waiting to hear. It doesn't matter, we'll love her anyway.' I won't say things have been easy, but I don't regret having her now, although of course sometimes I wish she had been normal.

The risk of having a Down's Syndrome

baby does increase with the mother's age. At the age of twenty, a woman has nearly a one-in-2000 chance of having an affected child. At the age of 30 this has risen to one in about 900; by 35, one in 365. At 37–38 it is around one in 200, and by 40 about one in 100. After this it rises still more steeply, so that a mother of 43 has a one-in-50 chance and a mother of 47 a one-in-20 chance. By the age of 50 the risk is about one in ten. There is also evidence that the risk of having a Down's Syndrome baby increases if the father is over 55.

Maternal age	Risk of Down's Syndrome
20	1/1923
21	1/1695
22	1/1538
23	1/1408
24	1/1299
25	1/1205
26	1/1124
27	1/1053
28	1/990
29	1/935
30	1/885
31	1/826
32	1/725
33	1/592
34	1/465
35	1/365
36	1/287
37	1/225
38	1/177
39	1/139
40	1/109
41	1/85
42	1/67
43	1/53
44	1/41
45	1/32
46	1/25
47	1/20
48	1/20
49	1/12

Table 3. Risk of having a liveborn child with Down's Syndrome by one year maternal age intervals from ages 20–49 years.

Neural tube defects

Neural tube defects, which include spina bifida and anencephaly, occur in about three in every 1000 live births. Early in pregnancy, a groove appears down the baby's back and this develops into the brain and spinal cord. Normally the groove closes into a tube in which the spinal cord and brain develops but in rare cases the tube does not close properly. If the defect is in the part of the tube that forms the brain, anencephaly results; this is always fatal as the upper skull and brain do not form. If the defect is lower down, then part of the spinal cord and nerves protrude, covered by a fragile membrane; the baby is usually paralysed from this point down. Sometimes, however, spina bifida can be less severe, is not visible from outside and results in minimal handicap.

As many as 85 per cent of babies severely affected with spina bifida also have a defect called hydrocephaly. Cerebro-spinal fluid accumulates in the head, causing mental retardation if untreated. Nowadays the fluid can be drained away after birth and surgery can repair the opening in the spine to reduce the risk of infection. Surgery and other techniques have improved the outlook for children suffering from this handicap.

Spina bifida can probably be largely prevented by an adequate diet before and during early pregnancy. Evidence has shown that taking vitamin supplements rich in B-group vitamins and folic acid has greatly reduced the incidence of spina bifida, even in mothers at greater risk because the handicap is in their family.

Cleft lip and palate

This is one of the most common abnormalities, affecting about one in 1000 babies. The cleft is caused when the tissues which move together to form the face in very early pregnancy do not fuse, leaving a gap which can involve the lip alone, the palate, or both. The cleft can be on one or both sides of the face and varies in its seriousness. The vast majority of children with cleft lip or palate are normal in other respects, but sometimes it is found accompanying some other abnormality.

Cleft palate can cause quite serious feeding problems in the early months, as the baby is unlikely to be able to suck well. The child will have difficulties in speaking and also teeth are likely to be missing or malformed in the area of the cleft. Plastic surgery, however, can now be carried out so that the cleft is completely repaired, inside and out, by the time the child reaches maturity. Speech therapy and orthodontic work are usually required.

Although cleft lip and palate are correctable, it is very distressing to give birth to an affected child:

Our son was born with a double cleft palate and lip. When he was born it looked terribly disfiguring, because the middle of his upper lip and jaw were pushed forward, rather like a beak. He had terrible feeding problems; he couldn't suck, and had to be fed at first with a spoon. You can imagine how difficult this is with a hungry, crying baby whose every instinct is to suck.

He had to have a series of operations throughout his childhood and the end result is very good. But the emotional effects of stays in hospital and of looking different to other children are harder to deal with than the physical repairs.

Abnormalities in the digestive tract

Also relatively common and correctable defects are abnormalities in the digestive tract. These include a blockage of the entrance to the stomach, often accompanied by an oesophageal/tracheal fistula, where the windpipe and gullet are joined; and blockages at various points in the digestive tract, including an imperforate anus. All these are quite easily corrected by surgery and some can even be detected by ultrasound.

Detecting abnormalities

Some tests are now available to screen all mothers, and others are available for those mothers who are at higher risk of having a handicapped child. Some of these tests are offered to women routinely, others only to women over a certain age who are already known to be at risk either because of family history or because of previous difficulties with pregnancies. Most maternity hospitals will explain at the booking-in clinic what their procedure is and which tests they offer to women. If they don't, and you would like to know, ask which tests they offer and when they do them.

Screening tests include ultrasound scans, which are now performed routinely at sixteen weeks at many hospitals; a blood test which can detect raised levels of a substance called alphafetoprotein in the blood, which may indicate a neural tube defect; amniocentesis – taking a sample of the waters surrounding the baby which enables the chromosomes to be examined, showing up a chromosomal abnormality and incidentally showing the child's sex; and rarer techniques such as fetoscopy, where the baby can be examined through a tube inserted into the womb and chorionic villi sampling, a new experimental technique which may one day replace amniocentesis.

Ultrasound

Ultrasound consists of high-frequency sound waves which are bounced off the baby to give a photographic picture of the foetus. Unlike X-rays, which have much higher powers of penetration, ultrasound will show up soft tissues and thus can give a complete picture of the growing baby, and is a very useful diagnostic tool.

An ultrasound scan tends to be given to all women at around sixteen weeks of pregnancy in hospitals which have the equipment. If not, women who may be at special risk because of problems with a previous pregnancy, or who would like to have a scan, can often be referred to a hospital where it can be performed. The reason for the routine use of ultrasound is that the pregnancy can be very accurately dated at around sixteen weeks by measuring the circumference of the baby's head, and this is very useful in avoiding problems later if the mother is unsure of her dates and does not know when the baby is due. The scan can also locate the position of the placenta, which can shed light on any bleeding later in pregnancy, and can be used to check that the baby has no major physical abnormalities such as anencephaly or stunted limbs. Ultrasound can also show up congenital heart defects, kidney disease and other phaly or badly formed limbs. Ultra-if the mother is expecting twins.

There has been some controversy about the safety of ultrasound, which has caused concern to women who are not sure whether they should accept a routine scan. Ultrasound has now been in use for many years without any evidence of harmful effects to the baby. Recently, the Royal College of Obstetricians and Gynaecologists issued a report recommending no change in the policy of carrying out routine scans at 16–18 weeks of pregnancy. Seventy-two per cent of mothers in England and

Wales have routine scans and a further 13 per cent have a scan for medical reasons, so some 85 per cent of mothers will have at least one scan in the course of their pregnancy.

All the indications are that the benefits of having ultrasound outweigh any potential risk. Not least is the benefit of reassurance given to many women at seeing their baby is alive and well. Ultrasound can also be used later in the pregnancy to check that the baby is growing well should there be any reason for concern about this. However, not everyone is happy with the experience of ultrasound:

Towards the end of my pregnancy they started to worry about whether my baby was growing properly. I don't know what started it all off, but once they'd got this idea into their heads they wouldn't leave me alone. I was in and out of hospital having blood pressure taken and having ultrasound scan after scan. My blood pressure was up – no doubt with all the worry – and they couldn't decide what to do. They said that they would have to induce the baby early to make sure that all would be well and then they changed their minds and decided to wait. I was in hospital for the last few weeks of the pregnancy and, of course, the baby decided to be late. They let me go two weeks overdue and then they decided to induce the birth, and by then I was so desperate I said, 'Yes.' It was a terrible birth ending with an emergency Caesarian, and when he was born he was seven pounds one ounce. Nor did he look overdue. I asked the consultant later, 'So what happened about this small baby?' There was nothing wrong at all, all my worries had been for nothing. They said they couldn't explain it but he had appeared small on the scan. So much for all their wonderful technology!

Some women – and doctors and midwives, too – feel that, with the increased reliance on new technology, many of the old skills in obstetrics are being lost:

I had shared care and I noticed a tremendous difference between my visits to the hospital and my visits to my very experienced GP. At the hospital people seemed to poke and probe for a long time and suggested that I might have another scan to check the baby was growing OK. When I went to my GP she examined me very quickly and said, 'Oh, this baby's doing fine, I should think he weighs about four pounds now.' I asked how she knew and she just said, 'Experience.' It seems that in hospitals you only see the young junior staff and the consultants are just called out for special occasions; no wonder you don't always get the best care and they give you all sorts of unnecessary tests.

Having an ultrasound scan

Having a scan is a simple procedure. In early pregnancy you are usually asked to drink a lot of water an hour or two before your appointment and not to empty your bladder. This pushes the womb up in the pelvis and will give the ultrasound operator a clearer view. You will be asked to lie down on a couch and remove any clothing that covers your abdomen. A cold jelly is then rubbed over the abdomen to enable the ultrasound operator to move the scanner smoothly over the area. As she does so, you will see the baby's outline appear on the television screen and you will also see the foetal movements. It can be quite difficult to interpret what you are seeing so, if you are not told, do ask. The operator can freeze the picture at any moment and point things out to you at length without exposing the baby to any more sound waves than are necessary. You will usually be able to see the baby's head, the arms and legs moving around, and some of the internal organs at work. You may even be able to see the baby sucking his thumb:

The woman took a lot of time to explain to me about what she was looking for and what she could see. I found all this terribly reassuring. She pointed out the heart beating, the cord and the placenta, the kidneys and the spine and showed me how much he was moving around.

Other women find the process unnerving especially if nothing is explained.

No one said anything to me and I was afraid to ask in case anything was wrong. She kept on looking at everything and taking measurements and I started to get very jumpy. Then she suddenly got up and said, 'I just want to get a second opinion on this' and I was terrified. I thought this is it, something's terribly wrong. I was in tears. Someone else came back and they were both looking at the screen, still not saying anything to me. 'What is it, what is wrong?' I finally asked. 'Nothing's wrong, I'm just checking these measurements.' I felt as if I wasn't a person, a mother, just a scientific toy.

Usually the baby's father is welcome to come and watch the process and see the baby on the screen. Many find this a very positive experience, as they are able to give support, but also the baby becomes real to them in an even more dramatic way than to the woman: 'It was hard for me to take in that she was pregnant until I saw the baby on the screen. It was fantastic – it made it come alive for me.'

Alphafetoprotein blood test

This test is a routine blood test carried out at between sixteen and eighteen weeks of pregnancy. It measures the level of a substance called alphafeto-protein (AFP) which gets into the mother's bloodstream from the baby. A high level of alphafetoprotein can mean a number of things: that the pregnancy is further advanced than was thought, that the mother is expecting twins, or that the baby is suffering from a neural tube defect. It can also mean nothing at all!

If a woman does have a higher than normal level of AFP, a second blood test will be done to confirm this. If this too is positive, then there is a roughly one-in-seven chance that the foetus has a neural tube defect. It is usually recommended that the woman have an ultrasound scan to check for the presence of anence-phaly or spina bifida. If all this is inconclusive, an amniocentesis is usually recommended so that the level of AFP in the amniotic fluid can be measured (see section below).

The problem with the AFP blood test is that the majority of women with a high AFP level will have an amniocentesis performed, accompanied by all the stress and worry involved, when there is actually nothing wrong with their baby. The chance of the level of AFP being high from other causes is greater than the risk of there being a neural tube defect.

Rather than performing the AFP test routinely without the mother being consulted, it might be better to explain what the test is for and what it entails and let the mother choose. Some people will welcome it, others prefer to do without:

> I had just had the scan, seen the baby moving, that its head was there and it was kicking its legs. I thought, we would have seen if there was anything really wrong, its head would have been the wrong shape or its legs paralysed. Anyway, I felt I couldn't possibly have aborted that baby once I I had seen him like that. So I decided not to have the test. What was the point of having it done when I could see there was nothing so very wrong with the baby and wouldn't have wanted an abortion anyway?

Further, not all neural tube defects are detected by the test. There is no absolute level of AFP in the amniotic fluid at which one can say, this baby is affected and this one isn't; an artificial line has to be drawn. If the level is set too high, more neural tube defects will be undetected. If it is too low, more women will have further tests with all the worry attached or even have an abortion when there is nothing wrong with their baby.

Some very recent information has shown that there may be a link between an abnormally low level of alphafeto-protein in the mother's blood and Down's Syndrome. This theory is now being tested, but if it were so it could be a wonderful screening test for women of all ages.

Amniocentesis

Amniocentesis (testing the waters) consists of taking a sample of the amniotic fluid surrounding the baby and analysing it. The amniotic fluid contains some of the baby's cells, and these can be cultured to show up any chromo-somal abnormalities. Amniocentesis can also be used to detect neural tube defects, as there will then be a very high level of AFP in the amniotic fluid; this is much more accurate than the AFP blood test.

Amniocentesis is usually offered to women over the age of 37 or 38, although policies differ from hospital to hospital and region to region. A survey carried out by the Maternity Alliance a few years ago showed that this test would be available to three-quarters of women over the age of 38. Most NHS doctors are reluctant to carry out the test before the age of 35, because there is only a one-in-300 chance of finding an abnormality at this age, while the chance of causing a miscarriage is about one in 150. By the age of 40, on the other hand, the chance of an abnormality has risen

to more than one in 100. If a consultant is unwilling to carry out the test despite a couple's worries, they can try asking a consultant who is more sympathetic to their viewpoint or, as a last resort, have it done privately at a cost of around £150 (in 1986-7).

The risk of miscarriage attached to amniocentesis is small, at around 1 – 1.5 per cent and there is some con-troversy as to whether this is a real risk at all, as no one understands why a miscarriage may occur or which women are at greater risk. However, for older mothers, especially those with a history of miscarriage or infertility and for whom a pregnancy is particularly precious, there is a real fear of inducing a miscarriage and this can make the decision to have an amniocentesis a very difficult one.

An amniocentesis is usually carried out at about sixteen weeks of pregnancy. This is the earliest time that sufficient amniotic fluid can be drawn off for testing. Amniocentesis is done on an out-patient basis, so you will not have to be admitted to hospital. Amniocentesis is almost always done now at the same time as an ultrasound scan. This is done first to establish that you are at least sixteen weeks pregnant and to see the exact position of the foetus and placenta. You are normally asked to have a full bladder for the scan and then to empty it before the amniocentesis is performed.

The needle is usually inserted without local anaesthetic, as the local anaes-thetic really only means you get two pin-pricks instead of one. The doctor directs the needle into the amniotic fluid and

Amniocentesis

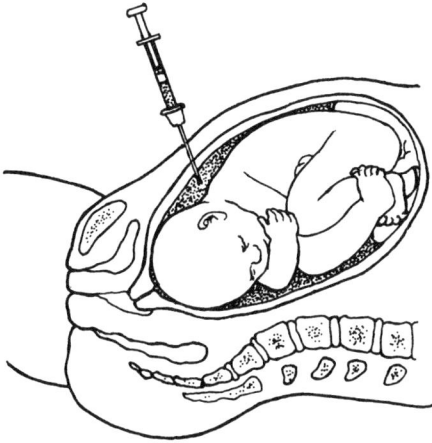

draws off about 30 millilitres of the pale yellow fluid. When ultrasound is used as well, the danger of the needle hitting the baby or placenta is very small. Most women do not find the procedure painful, and describe a slight cramp or pressure in the womb as the needle passes through the uterine wall. Some women feel a little sore for a day or two afterwards and you are usually advised to take it easy because of the slight risk of miscarriage. For some women, however, the test is not so straightforward:

We went along at 16-17 weeks; my husband came and we were all keyed up. They did the scan first and said the baby was lying all spread out so there were no big pockets of fluid to get the needle into, so it wasn't worth trying. We had to go back the following week - the anticlimax was awful. The second time they again said it wasn't very good, but because of pressure of time they'd better do it now; it would take three weeks to get the results at least, and if the sample

didn't 'take' we'd have to have another test. I found the process really quite unpleasant. They had to rake around to get enough fluid and I found that quite painful. Then I had a very low back pain which bothered me - the site of the injection didn't hurt at all. The discomfort, however, passed quickly - I lay on my side for half an hour afterwards and then felt fine.

Others find the process much easier than they thought:

It was very simple. I felt absolutely nothing. My husband was there and he said did you really not feel anything because they seemed to take pints of fluid! They were extremely helpful and reassuring and it was much, much easier than I had imagined it would be.

Once the test is done the fluid has to be sent off to be analysed. The cells in the fluid have to be cultured and grown over a couple of weeks, then crushed and looked at under a microscope so the chromosomes can be examined. Very occasionally the test fails and has to be repeated, two or three weeks further into the pregnancy:

I had an amnio at 16 weeks after much thought and consultation. The first one didn't take – and I had another at 20 weeks by which time I had felt the baby moving. I couldn't understand what was wrong with the first test and worried that it meant that something was wrong with the baby.

The fluid is also tested for high levels of alphafetoprotein which indicates the presence of a neural tube defect.

If you are the possible carrier of a genetic disease then tests can be carried out to identify up to 70 or 80 hereditary diseases. These tests are very time-consuming and expensive, so they will only be done if there is a history of an inherited illness which can be tested for in your family.

Waiting for the results can be the most difficult aspect of the whole procedure. Usually, women are told that the results will take three weeks, though sometimes it is sooner and rarely later: 'They said the results would take three weeks but in fact it was only two. They had tried to ring but we were out so they wrote us a very nice letter saying all was well.'

You are usually informed by letter or by telephone; you can telephone if the results are overdue. You can also ask to know the sex of the baby if you want to, though some hospitals insist on talking this over with you first:

> We had asked to know the sex of the baby but they were actually quite reluctant that we should know. They said go home and think about it, and asked probing questions about did we want a girl or boy. When they rang up to say the results were fine they didn't volunteer the information but we pressed it and they said it was a girl. We didn't really mind the sex, but we both had a slight preference for a girl. We were delighted and it was wonderful to know, which I hadn't in my earlier pregnancies. In

fact, knowing was one of the most important parts of the pregnancy.

There is some evidence that people who desperately want either a son or daughter have problems adjusting to the baby if they know in advance that it is the 'wrong' sex. In the heat of the birth itself, most parents are so pleased to know the baby is all right that they do not mind so much about its sex and the baby is there to love and care for. Knowing while pregnant, however, gives a parent time to brood over the as yet unknown person and sometimes to reject the baby, making it more difficult to adjust when the baby arrives.

This is a very individual matter, and people hold very different attitudes:

> Of course I wanted to know. I thought if it was there, in my notes, and other people knew, then of course I had the right to know.

> I asked them don't tell me! I didn't want to know, it would have spoiled it all, like unwrapping a present before your birthday.

> If it's a first baby, I think once you know you feel rather sad in any case, because you want both, you can't really decide which is your preference. So when they said it's a girl, I felt sad in a way that it wasn't a boy, though it wasn't that I actually wanted a boy.

Most hospitals will respect people's wishes in the matter although some will provide limited counselling to help a couple decide whether they want to know or not. Occasionally one partner wants to know the sex and the other doesn't; this is very hard to deal with. If one partner is told and hides it from the other, it casts a considerable strain over a relationship at a time when a couple should be as close and open with one another as possible.

Fetoscopy

This technique involves passing a very small tube containing a light and a lens into the womb so that the developing baby can be seen. The tube is introduced through a small incision made just above the pubic bone under a local anaesthetic. Fetoscopy is carried out in the second three months of pregnancy and samples of the baby's blood, skin and liver can be taken. A number of abnormalities can be detected by fetoscopy that could not be found out any other way, and it has recently been used to 'operate' on the unborn baby, allowing drugs and transfusions to be given directly into the baby's bloodstream.

The baby is usually viewed at around sixteen weeks and blood samples taken between seventeen and twenty-two weeks. External defects to the face or limbs, and neural tube defects are clearly visible. Haemophilia and other blood disorders can be detected, as can some diseases of the metabolism. The technique is not used lightly, however, as there is a substantially increased risk of miscarriage, death of the baby in the womb or premature labour.

Chorionic villi sampling

This is a relatively new technique which is now being tested in various hospitals as an alternative to amniocentesis. The great advantage of the test is that it can be carried out much earlier than amniocentesis, at around 8-10 weeks. This gives the mother who finds that her baby is abnormal the chance of an earlier abortion which can be carried out simply, rather than induced labour after she has felt the baby moving.

The CVS test is carried out by passing a thin tube through the cervix (neck of the womb) and removing a tiny fragment of tissue from the placenta. This can be done without an anaesthetic and, as with amniocentesis, ultrasound is used to show the exact position of the foetus and placenta. The vagina is cleaned with some antiseptic solution beforehand to prevent germs being introduced into the womb.

The test is not painful, but it is uncomfortable for many women, rather like having a cervical smear taken or, some women say, like having an IUD (contraceptive coil) fitted. The test takes about 10-20 minutes and you will be able to go home after about an hour. As with amniocentesis, you may be advised to take things easy for a day or two because of the risk of miscarriage. At the moment, this risk seems to be about one in 50, two or three times more likely than with amniocentesis. It is hard to be sure at present, however, when the test has not been in use for long and when there are not many doctors trained and skilled in performing it.

Chorionic villi sampling detects any chromosomal abnormalities as does amniocentesis, but it will not show up neural tube defects. Women who have this test will therefore also be given the AFP blood test to detect spina bifida.

If something goes wrong

The vast majority of women who have these screening tests in pregnancy find reassurance that all is well, and this enables them, and older mothers in particular, to relax and enjoy the rest of their pregnancy, free from unnecessary anxiety. It is worth mentioning, however, that none of the tests – not even amniocentesis – can absolutely guarantee a normal, perfect baby. They do not pick up all abnormalities, and sometimes problems can occur at the birth which handicap a child. The tests do, however, remove certain areas of worry from the parents' minds.

In the very small number of cases where an abnormality is found, however, the pregnancy is transformed from a happy event into a nightmare. Some women feel it is just as traumatic as losing a full-term baby, and the experience of knowing you are carrying a handicapped child and deciding whether to have a termination is one of the most difficult choices anyone can have to face. Often, too, hospitals are lacking in adequate support services and do not know how to deal with a couple's distress and grief. There is an organization. Support After Termination for Abnormality (SAFTA) which can help (see useful addresses). Outsiders may not understand or be able to sympathize. Doctors often do not explain the news well, or fail to see that the couple are not absorbing the information properly because they are so stricken with grief or shock:

The whole process was a disaster. They didn't ring up with the results of the amnio so in the end I rang them. They said, 'Oh yes, we can't discuss that over the phone, you must make an appointment to come in and see the consultant.' I knew then that something was wrong and I said, 'What's wrong? Is it Down's Syndrome?' She said no, it wasn't, but she couldn't say any more, she'd make an appointment. So we had to wait for the next day. They told us that there was a high level of AFP in the fluid and that it was likely the baby had spina bifida, and they would like to do another scan to check as they hadn't picked it up before. This time they did. They all looked at the screen, not me, although there were tears pouring down my face all the time. The consultant explained what the outlook was; that the majority of babies with this severe defect die soon after birth, that some can be operated on but would be permanently paralysed, and filled in this dismal picture for the child. We decided on an abortion straight away, but there had to be a few days wait for some beaurocratic reason. I was given no support, no counselling, nothing. There must be better ways of going about it.

A study carried out in the USA by the National Institutes for Child Health shows that of parents who discover that their baby is abnormal, 95 per cent decide on a termination. The figure is probably similar in Britain. Some hospitals advise that if a couple know they do not want a termination – they should not have the tests, to spare them 'unnecessary' expense. However, not all couples know till the decision is upon them and others feel they have the right to know in any case so that they can prepare themselves – both in a practical sense and from the emotional point of view:

I was 40 and had had years of infertility problems, in fact had been told I would never conceive a couple of months before I did. We discussed the possibility of a handicapped child and decided to have an amnio, because we didn't want to cope with a handicapped baby. But when we had the scan and had decided on a termination if anything was wrong before the amnio was carried out, when we actually saw the baby, we both came out and said, 'This is it, we won't have a termination.' But we still went ahead and had the amnio.

We would never have had a termination, I don't believe it's right. But if it had been a Down's Syndrome or something, I would have wanted to know so we could prepare ourselves, read up about it, tell the family in advance. I don't see why they should keep that from you.

It is a particularly harrowing experience if the mother is carrying a sex-linked genetic disease which affects only boys, such as haemophilia or Duchenne muscular dystrophy. The latter is a particularly distressing disease in which a child who appears normal at birth suffers a gradual loss of muscular strength, becomes progressively para-lysed and finally dies at the age of twenty.

If the mother is known to be carrying the disease, there is a 50 per cent chance that a boy will have the disease. Amniocentesis can tell the parents the child's sex, but not whether he has the disease, so parents can be faced with the agonizing choice of terminating the pregnancy if they are carrying a boy, without knowing if he would be affected or not. A girl will stand a 50 per cent chance of being a carrier, but will not have the disease.

The existence of these tests does help many women enjoy their pregnancy free of certain worries but it also presents some very difficult choices. Some women feel they can only embark on a pregnancy in later life because they have the option of discovering if the baby has a chromosomal abnormality, while others feel uncertain:

We agreed we couldn't have coped with a severely handicapped baby and had all the tests. But I don't think the tests being available influenced my decision to have a baby. Having a baby is a very emotional decision. I was glad to have the tests but I didn't really think about it in advance – I would have taken the risk.

Other mothers regret the existence of such tests, as they feel it puts an extra strain on the pregnancy:

As I was 38 when my first baby was conceived, I decided I would have the amniocentesis done. In fact, this turned the first six months of my pregnancy, a time which should have been a happy one for me, into a nightmare.

First I refused to 'bond' with the baby in my mind, in case there was something wrong with him or her. By the time the test was to be done, I had worked myself into quite a state about it, and convinced myself that the result would be a bad one.

When the test was done I felt contractions as if I was starting labour which terrified me; later I had a threatened miscarriage, which I'm sure was connected. I heard sooner than I expected, but it was neither a positive nor a negative result, as the test hadn't taken. They said there was just time to repeat the test if I wanted, and after a great deal of agonizing I decided to do this.

Again I had to wait two weeks – in fact a little more – before the result came. All was clear, and I felt a great relief. But the whole business made me feel enormously protective towards my baby, not wanting him to be interfered with and, at the same time, alienated all that time from him in case he was abnormal.

Because amniocentesis can only be carried out at 16-18 weeks, and the results take two to four weeks to come back, a woman can be as much as 22 weeks pregnant when she knows that her baby is abnormal. This means that she will have felt the baby move and that she will be having an abortion almost at the time when the baby could live if it were born prematurely. The abortion will be a proper labour, although the baby is killed first by the injection of saline solution or another substance into the womb. Labour may well last a long time and many women find the experience of labour without the reward at the end a terrible experience:

> I couldn't bear to think about it or talk about it. It was a travesty of everything I'd ever read about the glory and wonder of childbirth. It was agony, and I just wanted to be doped until it was all over. I wouldn't let my husband be there, I couldn't have borne it for him to have to suffer it too.

Although choosing to have a termination is a terrible and shocking experience, those couples who do so find this preferable to bringing a severely handicapped child into the world. However, there are couples who do choose to bring up their handicapped children, or adopt other people's, and find great rewards in doing so:

> Of course we found it hard at first having a Down's baby, and we've had hard times since he was born, but in the end we just loved him – he's our child and he's brought a lot of love into our lives.

CHAPTER FIVE

Having the Baby

Tremendous changes have taken place in childbirth methods in hospitals over the last decade or so and mothers are given an increasing amount of choice in how they want to have their babies. Making a choice, however, means finding out what the options are and understanding what labour, both normal and with complications, involves.

Labour is divided into three clear stages. The first stage is when the muscles of the womb contract increasingly powerfully, pulling open the cervix or neck of the womb to allow the baby's head to come through. The second stage is when you push with the contractions to force the baby out of the womb, and it ends with the birth of the baby. The third stage is the expulsion of the placenta or afterbirth.

How labour begins

Every labour is different for every woman, and that is why it is so difficult for those who have never had a baby to find out what the experience is likely to be like. Labour begins in a number of different ways. Sometimes the first sign is a 'show' – you will see the blood-tinged, gelatinous plug that has sealed the entrance to the womb come away. In some women, the waters break first – this can result in a dramatic gush of fluid or it can simply be a slow leak. If the waters leak for more than 24 hours without labour getting well under way it is advisable to contact the doctor or midwife, as once the waters have broken the baby is exposed to infection.

The most common sign that labour is beginning is a cramp-like pain, rather like the onset of the menstrual period, in your lower abdomen or back. You will probably soon feel this pain turn into distinct contractions, which you can feel as a tightening and hardening of the abdomen accompanied by growing discomfort or pain. These contractions differ from the contractions felt throughout the pregnancy only in their greater intensity. As labour progresses, the contractions become stronger and closer together and also last a little longer.

The duration of the early part of

labour varies enormously – some women find the contractions continue without becoming too painful for hours or even days. Others find that they build up very rapidly. You are usually asked to report at the hospital when the contractions are about five minutes apart; however, you will know how long it takes you to get to the hospital and you will not want to be travelling if the contractions are very strong and you are in great discomfort, so go when you are ready. Many women prefer to spend the early part of labour at home in familiar surroundings, able to wander around and make a cup of tea and feel that everything is normal. Indeed, the stress of going into hospital too soon has been known to stop a labour which has not got properly underway. If you are having your baby at home, or a 'domino' delivery, you will want to phone the midwife as soon as you are sure labour is established.

When you arrive at the hospital the midwife will take some notes, time your contractions, feel your abdomen and listen to the baby's heart-beat and then give you an internal examination to see how far your cervix has dilated. This is usually measured in centimetres; half dilation is five centimetres or so and full dilation is approximately ten centimetres. Some midwives will talk of 'two fingers' dilated – a finger is about equal to a centimetre. Often it takes a lot longer to dilate the first few centimetres than the last, as the contractions at the beginning of labour are not so strong. Some women, especially those who have had babies before, find that they are already well dilated without knowing it

when they arrive at the hospital.

Many women find internal examinations during labour very uncomfortable. Make sure they are done as soon as one contraction is over so that you are not actually being examined during a contraction. It is important that the midwife can check how your labour is progressing. If you find an internal too uncomfortable lying on your back, ask the doctor or midwife if she or he can examine you lying on your side.

When you arrive at the hospital your baby's heart-beat will usually be routinely monitored with an external monitor; this is tied around your tummy with a strap and you will be asked to keep still so your movements do not interfere with the reading. Most women find this very restricting, but it is helpful to know that the baby is all right. If all is well, the monitor will be removed after 20 or 30 minutes – it may be replaced again at some point in the labour just to check that the baby is not distressed.

It is a good idea to tell the staff when you arrive if you have any strong feelings about the way you want the labour conducted. Once it has really got underway, you may find yourself swept along by events. Most hospitals today are aware that women should be given a choice about pain relief and about the position they would like to adopt to deliver the baby. Also raise any queries about episiotomies, clamping and cutting the cord, anything else you wish to know and any other worries you may have. Ideally you will have discussed this with staff beforehand and any strong views recorded in your notes.

Special risks for the older mother

Many older women do fear that child-birth will be much riskier for them than for younger women, and riskier for the baby, too. This is true, but it is not that much riskier. Modern hospital care and antenatal screening reduce a lot of the risks, and a mother in her late thirties who is fit and healthy, eats well and takes care of herself in pregnancy is likely to do as well or better than a younger woman who has not taken care of herself. Woman under twenty are also at greater risk. The number of children you have had and the spacing between them is important too: the risks for the first and fourth or more births are greater than for second or third births, and the risks go up if you have a baby within two years of the previous delivery. If you have had a child before, it doesn't matter how long ago this was; a second birth is still likely to be quicker and easier.

Part of the greater risk of pregnancy and childbirth for the older mother is due to the fact that she is more likely to suffer from diabetes, cardiovascular disease and other illnesses which affect pregnancy. The risk of hypertension for older mothers increases by about 50 per cent. The risk of pre-eclampsia, haemorrhage following birth and dysfunctional labour (when the cervix does not dilate properly) are more prevalent in women over 35. The incidence of placenta praevia, when the placenta is situated over the entrance to the womb and can therefore come away and cause haemorrhage before or during the birth, or other forms of antepartum haemorrhage, increases with age and with the number of pregnancies – for first-time mothers the risk goes up from 3 per cent for under 25s to 5 per cent for over 35s, and doubles for mothers having a fourth child. There is also a small increased risk in prematurity for infants of women aged 35-44, but this is only slightly higher than for infants of mothers in their twenties and thirties. There is also, of course, a greater risk of having an abnormal baby, but this can now usually be screened for early in pregnancy (see Chapter Four). The greater risk of miscarriage for older mothers may be linked to a higher number of abnormal embryos being conceived.

However, it may be true that the higher incidence of dysfunctional labour, Caesarian section and other problems may be caused by obstetric intervention in the older mother. If this baby is a more precious one because of previous in-fertility problems or because the mother is unlikely to conceive again, then doctors are inclined to intervene on behalf of the baby at a slightly greater risk to the mother. There is an increased risk that if the baby is overdue, the placenta of an older woman will fail sooner than of a woman in her twenties and fail to nourish the baby properly, so a birth is more likely to be induced. Induction means that labour is more likely to be intensely painful, necessita-ting pain relief and further intervention. It is also likely to be linked to dys-functional labour, because the cervix is not yet ready to dilate. The higher rate of Caesarian section is probably linked more to caution on the part of doctors than to any substantial increase in the real risk to mother or baby.

Statistics show that forceps deliveries and Caesarian sections are more common among older mothers. In 1980 in England and Wales, for those having their first baby, just under 20 per cent of women under 25 had forceps deliveries, compared with 29 per cent of women aged 25–34 and 33 per cent of women over 35. The risk of having a Caesarian section for older mothers having their first baby, however, is much greater; only 8 per cent of such mothers under 25 had Caesarians compared with 12 per cent of women aged 25–34 and over 30 per cent of women over 35. Curiously, older mothers seem less likely to end up with episiotomies. While 70 per cent of women under 25 having their first baby had episiotomies and 72 per cent of women aged 25–34, just under 60 per cent of first-time mothers over 35 had one. However, this may be simply because more had Caesarian sections!

There is some controversy as to whether older mothers have longer labours than younger women. Some obstetricians have said that they have observed that women over 35 tend to have longer labours, but in 1980 20 per cent of mothers over 35, having first babies, had long labours compared with 16 per cent aged 25–34 and 10 per cent aged under 25. This is not an enormous difference.

The other risks faced by older mothers are risks to the baby. Women over 35 have about three times the risk of having a miscarriage and about twice the risk of losing their baby before, during or after the birth. The increased risk of having a premature or low birth-weight baby probably accounts for part of this, as does the increased risk of having an abnormal child. However, some of these risks are linked to conditions which the mother will know about in advance of the baby being born. The healthy, fit, well-nourished mother who suffers no illnesses is not likely to be at much more risk of losing her baby than a woman having a baby in her twenties.

Pain relief in labour

The pain of labour is very different from other kinds of pain; it is the pain of your body doing a very hard and laborious job, not the pain of your being in any way harmed or damaged. However, labour is normally a very painful experience. Many people have tried to gloss around this or give the impression, that properly prepared and armed with breathing exercises and the right attitude, you will not feel pain; this means that many women are taken by surprise and feel that they have failed when they do experience intense pain in labour and feel that they need some relief from it. It is known that fear and tension can create additional pain in labour and make it intolerable. If you tense all your muscles and fight the contractions, you will make it much more difficult for your body to do its job. You need to think, therefore, of helping your body through the contractions. This thinking is behind the various techniques of breathing and preparation which are taught to women in antenatal classes during pregnancy. By accepting the pain and dealing with it, many women find that they do not need pain-killing drugs which might also interfere with their being in control. For others experiencing a long and difficult labour, pain-killing drugs may provide much needed relief.

Breathing techniques

Slow, deep breathing will help you to relax between, and at the beginning and end of, contractions. At the height of a contraction, it may help to breath quickly and lightly, taking air into the top part of your lungs only. During the transition between the first and second stages, when you may feel the desire to push the baby out the midwife may ask you to wait till she is sure the cervix is fully dilated - very short, rapid, panting breaths may help you to overcome the desire to push.

Pain-relieving drugs

There are a number of drugs available which can be given to women in labour to relieve pain. They are particularly useful if you are experiencing a very long labour, if the baby is presenting the wrong way (see below) or if you are becoming exhausted. These drugs, however, can pass into the baby's bloodstream and affect the baby, or may affect the progress of the labour. Many women find it useful to wait a little between the moment they first feel that they may want pain relief and deciding to accept it. In the meantime, they may find that the labour is progressing very well and that they are nearly ready for the baby to be born. If the progress is slow, however, or there is any problem, they can still decide to accept some pain relief.

Gas and air

Nitrous oxide (laughing gas) mixed with oxygen can be very useful at the peak of labour, and it has the advantages that it does not affect the baby, and also that you administer it yourself. The gas and air is contained in a large canister and you will be given a mouthpiece or mask through which to inhale it. The idea is that you can breathe it in a minute or so before the height of a contraction to help you through the most intense part. You may feel very light-headed when you breath it in, but this will pass as soon as you stop. Some women, however, do not like the 'woozy' sensation it gives them, while others feel ill or are very sick.

Pethidine

This drug, a synthetic equivalent to morphine, acts as a relaxant and relieves anxiety and thus pain; however, not all women find it is an effective form of pain relief. Some find that it makes them feel heavy and out of control without helping the pain much. Pethidine crosses the placenta and can affect the baby, making it drowsy at birth, especially if the drug is given close to delivery - it should be given at least two hours before the baby is born. Some babies even need resuscitation. Pethidine can also make the mother feel sick.

Epidural anaesthesia

An epidural consists of a local anaesthetic which completely numbs the abdomen and legs, thus removing all sensation of contractions. If an epidural is timed just right, it can be allowed to wear off for the second stage so that you can feel and push with each contraction, thus helping the baby out. It has no effect on the baby, but the problem is that because some women cannot feel anything they cannot participate in the second stage of labour, which is likely to be prolonged, and the baby is more likely then to be delivered with forceps. The 1977 National Epidural Survey showed that 70 per cent of mothers who had epidurals for their first birth, and 40 per cent of mothers in second births, ended up with forceps.

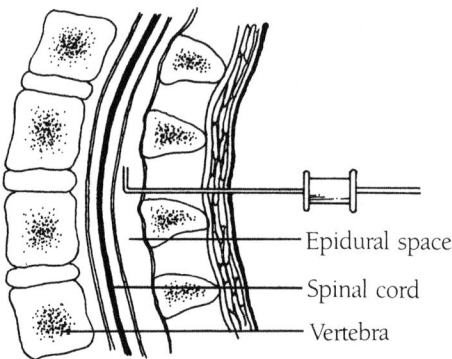

Epidural space
Spinal cord
Vertebra

An epidural is injected into the epidural space in the spine between the vertebrae and the membrane enclosing the spinal cord. You will be asked to lie on your left side, pulling your legs up to make as tight a ball as possible to make it easier for the anaesthetist to put the needle into the spine. You will be given a local anaesthetic so you do not feel the tube being inserted; the anaesthetic is then put in. You will feel it like a cold fluid

running down your legs. The catheter is left in your back so the epidural can be 'topped up'; you will also normally have a catheter put in to empty your bladder as you will not be able to do this yourself, and a drip set up in case your blood pressure should suddenly fall, as can happen with an epidural.

For some women, an epidural is the answer to a difficult labour:

> I had been in labour for hours, with very strong contractions, but I simply wasn't dilating much. Eventually I was exhausted and felt I couldn't take any more. They offered me an epidural, and I reluctantly accepted. I must say that the effect was wonderful; within a few minutes of them putting it in I was sitting up and chatting to the nurses and felt that I could cope again.

Epidurals can cause problems, however. In one in five occasions the epidural does not take properly and provides inadequate pain relief. Occasionally – one in 100 cases – the needle punctures the membrane enclosing the spinal cord; this means that you are more heavily anaesthetized and can suffer headaches which can last up to a week after the birth. Very rarely, in about 1 in 100,000 cases, permanent damage can result.

> I hated it. First the anaesthetist had trouble getting it in and in fact a bit of plastic tube broke off and is still floating around somewhere in my spine. Then I had all these tubes and drips set up, and I couldn't get up and walk for hours after the birth. I didn't feel or see the baby born at all because

I could feel nothing; I had no idea it would be like that. What's more, because I couldn't push, he was delivered by forceps so now I have all the pain of lots of stitches which I would rather have done without.

Women having an epidural should be aware that they are often starting off a chain of medical intervention which they might otherwise have done without. On the other hand, if the labour is likely to be a very difficult one, it means that you are spared a lot of pain and are already anaesthetized if the baby has to be delivered by forceps. And if you should need an emergency Caesarian, the epidural will enable you to be awake and avoid a general anaesthetic when your baby is born.

Pudendal block

This is a pain-killing injection given in the vaginal wall with a special needle if a high forceps delivery is necessary, so that you will feel no pain at all.

Local anaesthetics are also given if an episiotomy is done and for any stitching done afterwards.

Difficult labours

Normally the baby is born with the head down, facing backwards so that the widest part of the baby's head passes down through the widest part of the pelvis. The baby's head pressing down on the cervix helps it to dilate, and the baby rotates as it is born, helping the body slip out behind the head.

Some babies, however, are born in a different position, and this normally causes problems in labour. A posterior presentation means that the baby faces forwards; its spine can press against the mother's as it moves down, causing pain and slowing up labour, and because the widest part of the baby's head is passing through the narrowest part of the pelvis the baby can more easily get stuck here, again prolonging labour and sometimes necessitating forceps.

A breech birth occurs when the baby does not turn, so that the head is not born first; breech babies are normally born buttocks first, occasionally feet first. About four births in a hundred are breech. Most breech births are straightforward, though you are most likely to need intervention, especially in a first birth. Many women are advised to have an epidural; usually the baby's head is delivered with forceps to protect it, and you are likely to have an episiotomy anyway to help the baby's head out. If you should need an emergency Caesarian, the epidural will already be set up.

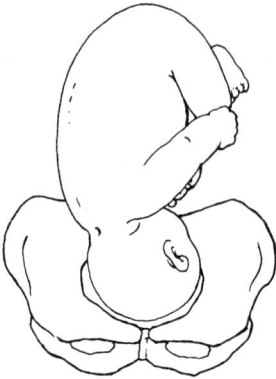

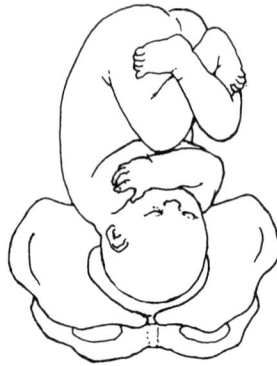

| Right occipito anterior (normal) | Right occipito posterior | Breech |

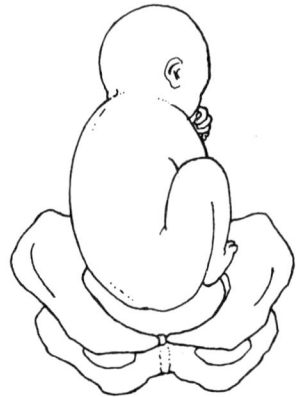

Medical intervention

Over the past decade or two hospitals have increasingly used a variety of techniques which have revolutionized the process of childbirth. Most of these are intended to save lives, and frequently they do. However, many interventions have become routine in some hospitals, thus interfering with the birth process in many mothers who are not at risk. Hospitals are now more likely to discuss any possible intervention with you, and you should make your views clear, although obviously everyone should accept that intervention may be necessary in case of an emergency.

Episiotomy

An episiotomy is a small incision made in the perineum, the skin between the vagina and the anus, to enlarge the vaginal opening and help the delivery of the baby's head. The cut is made with scissors under a local anaesthetic when the baby's head comes into view. Done properly, the perineum will have stretched very thin and the cut can be made with the minimum of damage and bleeding. An episiotomy should not be necessary in a normal delivery, and you can ask not to have one if you prefer.

Episiotomy

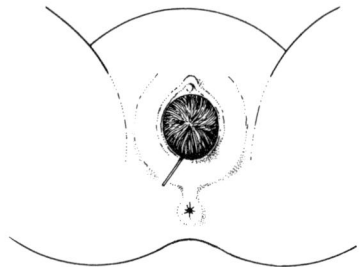

However, there is some controversy over whether it is better to have a small episiotomy or risk tearing when the baby's head is born. Some feel that a small tear is better and heals more rapidly, others that it is easier to sew up a clean cut. You can certainly ask that you are sewn up afterwards by a skilled doctor rather than an unskilled trainee. You should not feel the stitches; if you do, ask to have a local anaesthetic.

Induction

This is an artificial starting off of labour if it fails to start when all the indications are that the baby is overdue or if there is some need to deliver the baby early. Normally you will not be allowed to go much more than two weeks past your due date if the dates are firm and have been confirmed by ultrasound, as there is some risk that the placenta will not be functioning so well. This is a particular risk in older mothers. Tests can be done to check that the placenta is working normally and you may also be asked to keep a record of the foetus' movements. If there is evidence that the baby is not growing well, that foetal movements are becoming infrequent or the mother is suffering from high blood pressure, then induction will almost certainly be recommended. Many women are by this time quite willing for the birth to be induced:

> The last few months of pregnancy I was in and out of hospital having tests. I had an agonizing pain under the ribs which I knew was caused by the baby but they wanted to check it wasn't something else. I felt incredibly tired – I couldn't cope with the pain and not sleeping, so they decided to induce the birth – I was happy that this was done. But when I turned up at the clinic they said you're too tired to cope with labour now – go home, rest for a week, don't do anything,

and if the baby doesn't come we'll induce it next week.

Labour can be started artifically in several ways. The membranes containing the waters can be broken artificially if the baby is overdue or near to term; this will usually start labour, but if it doesn't other intervention will be needed as there is a risk of infection once the waters have been broken if the baby isn't delivered within 24 hours. An artificial rupture of the membranes (ARM) or amniotomy is performed with an instrument like a long crochet hook. This should be quite painless. The technique is also used to speed up labour, as, once the waters have broken, the baby's head, unprotected by the bag of waters, presses harder against the cervix, encouraging the uterus to contract. The contractions will become much stronger and you will also feel some of the waters gushing out with each contraction.

Prostaglandin pessaries can also be used to start off labour. These are usually inserted into the vagina where the effect of the hormones close to the cervix is to trigger labour. A man's sperm contains prostaglandin, which is why women at risk of a premature birth should avoid full sexual intercouse and why one of the best natural ways to induce labour is to make love. A prostaglandin-induced labour works very well because, once started, labour can proceed without any further intervention.

If labour does not start in any other way, an oxytocin drip is used. Oxytocin is the hormone which naturally causes the contractions of labour and various artificial forms of it can be used. A drip is inserted into your arm – you can ask that it is put into the arm you use least and that you have a long tube connecting you to the drip so that you can move around and change position as much as possible. The contractions caused when you are on an oxytocin drip are usually stronger, longer and more painful, and you may also find that you are plunged into the height of labour without having time to adjust to gradually increasing contractions, which can make the pain more difficult to cope with. Pain relief is often found necessary in these circumstances, and this in itself can lead to further intervention.

Electronic foetal monitoring

The baby's heartbeat and the strength of your contractions can now be measured electronically. It can be very reassuring to be able to hear and actually see throughout the delivery that the baby is well and not in distress, although it can also be checked using an old-fashioned ear trumpet or stethoscope. The disadvantage of electronic foetal monitoring is that you will be attached to a machine during labour and you may feel that it is being paid more attention than you. You will not be free to move around, and sometimes the machines do not work properly. There is also evidence that the slightest change in the baby's heart-beat will cause intervention, which may not have been necessary. Some studies have shown that where electronic foetal monitoring has been carried out routinely, the number of Caesarians carried out rises dramatically, even though there was no evidence to show that these were necessary.

Monitoring can be done with an external monitor strapped to your abdomen. Most women find this very awkward as they have to keep still, and it has a tendency to slip off during a contraction: 'They kept fussing around and trying to put it back on and I couldn't concentrate on what I was doing. Most of the time it wasn't in the right place and you just heard a lot of noise, not the baby's heart-beat.'

An internal monitor works better and is less restricting for the mother. However, the waters must be broken and the cervix at least 2–3 centimetres dilated for this to be attached to the baby's head. A tiny scar like a pin-prick will be left after the monitor is removed but it is unlikely to cause the baby much discomfort.

Forceps

Forceps deliveries are carried out when the first stage has been carried out and the cervix is fully dilated, but for some reason the baby's head is not coming down the birth canal or if the baby is in distress and needs to be born rapidly. Premature babies may well be delivered by forceps to spare their heads from being too compressed as they come through the birth canal and forceps are also usually used to protect the baby's head in a breech birth.

If your baby needs a forceps delivery you will be asked to lie on your back and your legs will be put into stirrups. You will be given a local anaesthetic and an episiotomy will be done to increase the vaginal opening. The forceps will then be gently inserted around the baby's head and gentle pulling will help the head out. Once the head is born the rest of the delivery occurs normally. If the baby's head is facing the wrong way, then forceps may be used to rotate the baby's head to help delivery.

Forceps deliveries are very safe and there is little chance of the baby being harmed in any way, although most will have marks on the head from the forceps for a few days after the birth. Forceps deliveries occur more often after a protracted labour where the mother becomes exhausted, where she has had an epidural and cannot feel to push with each contraction, or where the baby's head is large or in the wrong position.

Sometimes a vacuum extractor, called a ventouse, is used instead of forceps. This is a cup attached to a vacuum pump which is placed on the baby's head. It can be used before the cervix is fully dilated and is used, in conjunction with the mother's pushing, to help the baby out. A small circular mark where the cup was placed will show on the baby's head for a few days after the delivery.

Caesarian section

Caesarian sections are carried out more frequently than ever before; about one in nine births in the UK is now by Caesarian. The main reason for this change is that the operation has become much safer than previously. Improvements in anaesthetics have lowered the risk, especially since a planned Caesarian can now be done with an epidural rather than general anaesthetic.

The development of the low, transverse 'bikini cut' incision also made the operation safer and more acceptable, and decreased the risk for women who may want to have a later birth the normal way.

A recent survey carried out by the organization Maternity Alliance, One Birth in Nine, which covered 80 per cent of maternity hospitals and one in five obstetricians, gave some disturbing reasons for the increase in the number of Caesarians. The major reasons given were to prevent the stillbirths and deaths of newborn babies by performing Caesarians for breech births, premature and low birth-weight babies and when the baby showed signs of distress. But doctors also said that Caesarians were given because staff were inexperienced in dealing with difficult vaginal deliveries.

The most common reason for a Caesarian is when the baby's head is too big to pass through the pelvis, but other

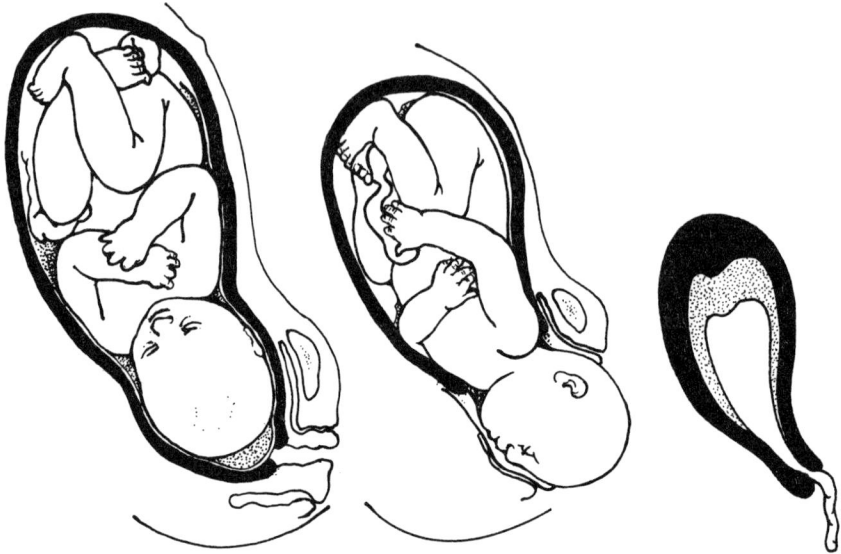

Normal labour: first stage   second stage   third stage

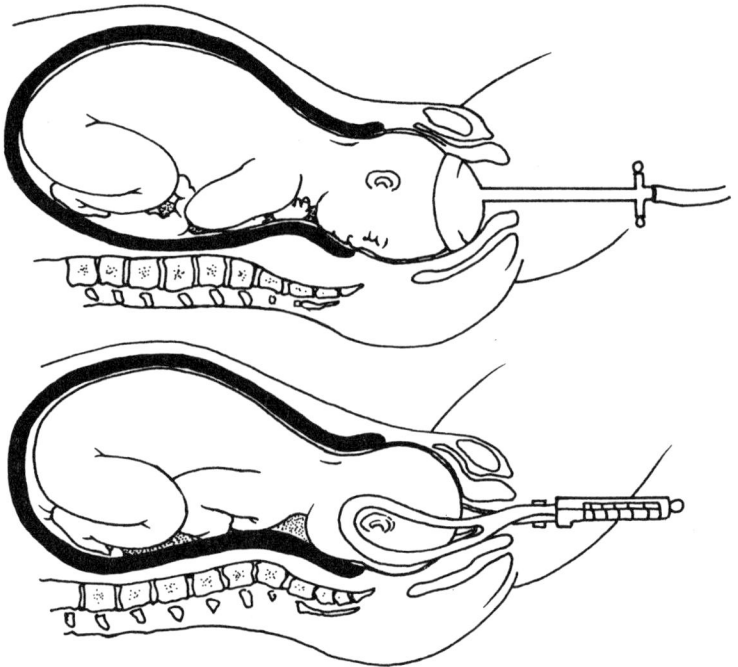

Assisted deliveries: ventouse (top) and forceps

reasons include when the mother is suffering from a disease like diabetes and chronic high blood pressure, or when the uterus does not contract properly, even with stimulation, or when the placenta is wrongly positioned (placenta praevia).

The mother's age will also be taken into account, as it is anticipated that older mothers will have more difficult labours and the baby may be more precious, especially if the woman has suffered infertility or miscarriages or may not conceive again. In these circumstances a doctor may prefer to do a Caesarian than take any risk for the baby:

> The staff never mentioned my age at all. I wasn't made to feel old. It was only at the end when they discovered she was breech that it suddenly came up, because they wanted me to have a Caesarian. They said, 'Well, it's your first baby, it's breech, you've had infertility problems and you're 40. This might be your only baby, so you want to be sure that nothing goes wrong.'

What happens during a Caesarian

If you know in advance that you are going to have a Caesarian, you can plan for it. You can choose to have the operation done under an epidural anaesthetic so that you can see and participate in the birth and see or hold your baby as soon as he is born. Your husband is also likely to be present for the whole of the operation. You can also make plans for the extra support you will need when you come out of hospital. If the operation is done as an emergency, however, you are likely to be given a general anaesthetic as setting up an epidural takes time. Your husband may not be able to be present and you are likely to suffer the after-effects of the anaesthetics, making it more difficult to bond with your new baby.

A Caesarian section usually takes about 45 minutes in all, although the baby is delivered in the first 5–10 minutes, the rest of the operation being the stitching up. The surgeon makes a cut about 12 centimetres long, usually horizontally and just below the bikini line. He or she then cuts horizontally through the lower part of the uterus, where there are no main blood vessels. The bag of waters may break of its own accord or have to be broken and the fluid is sucked away. The surgeon then puts his hands into the uterus and rotates the baby's head so that it appears in the incision. The baby is helped out with the hands or sometimes forceps, an assistant usually pushing on the top part of the uterus. An injection of ergometrine, a drug which makes the uterus contract and stops bleeding is given and the rest of the baby is brought out. The placenta is then delivered and the uterus is sewn up, then the abdominal wall.

Although the Caesarian section is a very safe operation, there is always a risk, albeit a slight one, in such surgery. Many women experience quite a lot of post-operative pain and may find that they cannot get comfortable for breast-feeding. Mothers often find it takes them longer to bond with their baby because they are feeling so rough in the days following the delivery:

> Having a Caesarian leaves you so incapacitated it takes so much longer to do things for the baby. Everything the baby does makes you feel so uncomfortable – lifting, feeding – and you are tied down with drips and bottles draining the wound for two days. Your mind is geared to you and not to the baby – it is harder to bond.
>
> Because of this I so much apprecia-ted the time I had with her at the beginning. The Caesarian was planned, so it was done with an epidural and I was awake. She was born onto me though I couldn't feel it – I was able to hold her straight away. I was able to think, 'this is my baby and no mistake', and the three of us had about one and a half hours together after the birth. Without that I think it would have been really hard.

The premature delivery

No one knows what causes a premature labour, nor can much be done to prevent it. There are drugs which can be given to try to stop labour, but the success rate is not very high and in any case these drugs may affect the baby. Multiple births are more likely to result in the birth of premature and low birth-weight babies, especially if the mother is having more than twins!

Prematurity is defined as much in terms of weight as actual age from conception. A distinction is made between babies who are of low birth weight although they are born at the right time – they are known as 'small-for-dates' – and babies who are born too early. About 6 or 7 per cent of babies are born weighing less than five and a half pounds (2500 grams) and these are responsible for a large proportion of infant deaths. All low birth-weight babies are likely to have problems in adjusting to life outside the womb and to need special care.

Babies are born 'small-for-dates' for a number of reasons. Sometimes the baby does not grow enough in the last months in the womb because the mother is malnourished, smokes or drinks a lot, suffers from pre-eclampsia or because the placenta is not working properly (placental insufficiency). Twins often do not grow as large as a single baby would, and some babies are small for genetic reasons or because they have some other abnormality. If the baby appears not to be growing well in the last month or so of pregnancy and the woman suffers from pre-eclampsia or placental insufficiency, the baby may be induced because it stands a better chance of survival once it has been born. No one really knows what triggers a premature birth, as the reasons why labour starts normally are very obscure. Research is being carried out into the reasons for premature delivery and also to find some effect-ive way of delaying labour if this will increase the baby's chances of survival.

However, enormous advances have

been made in the care of premature and low birth-weight babies and today they stand a much better chance of survival. In 1982, 40 per cent of babies weighing 1000 grams or less (2 lb.) survived, 83 per cent of babies weighing between 1000 and 1500 grams (2-3 lb.) survived, and 95 per cent of babies weighing 1500-2000 grams (3-4½ lb.) survived. Measured by gestational age, 70 per cent of babies born at 27 or 28 weeks survived, 80 per cent born at 29 weeks survive and over 30 weeks the vast majority will survive - all these figures, of course, applying to babies who are given special care immediately after birth. Tiny babies of as little as twenty weeks have been known to survive, although this is rare.

It is comforting to know that if your baby is born prematurely, but after the 28-week stage of pregnancy, he or she stands a good chance of survival. However, going into premature labour is an alarming and frightening experience. Most mothers are completely unprepared and fear that their baby will not survive. This may colour the whole birth process. The experience can be made worse by being in the wrong place:

George was born at 28 and a half weeks. We had been on holiday when my waters started to leak, so I went to the nearest cottage hospital where they really didn't have a clue about anything. We decided that we just had to get back to London where we could have the proper care - I was going to have him at one of the big teaching hospitals. I was in a terrible state of anxiety wondering if labour really would start and whether the baby could possibly survive. Once we got to London they said that they couldn't stop labour from happening because once the waters have gone the baby is liable to infection. It was my second birth and a normal labour, although I was advised not to have any pain relief as this would affect the baby and make his chances poorer.

He spent weeks in special care, coming home just before Christmas. I was terrified the whole time that he wouldn't make it, and in fact one of the other babies in the neonatal unit born at the same time as George died while we were there. It was terrible; I just kept thinking, 'that could be me, that could be me.'

Care of the premature baby

Premature babies are not yet ready to live in the environment outside the womb. The layer of fat under the skin has not yet been laid down, so the premature baby cannot control his body temperature. Many pre-term babies suffer from the respiratory distress syndrome. Their lungs do not contain enough of a substance called surfactant which is necessary for getting enough oxygen. The baby has to make an enormous effort to breathe and without help will rapidly become exhausted. Such babies will need to be given oxygen through a tiny tube through the nostrils or through a face mask; or a mechanical ventilator, which does the work of breathing for the baby, can be used.

Some low birth-weight babies have low blood sugar; this can also happen if the mother is diabetic or if the delivery was a difficult one. An intravenous drip may be set up to give the baby enough nourishment.

Many premature babies suffer from jaundice. About half of all babies develop mild jaundice, in fact, as a new-born baby has a surplus of red blood cells which are broken down after birth, producing a substance called bilirubin. The baby's liver sometimes cannot cope with the bilirubin rapidly enough and the baby becomes jaundiced. If a baby is very jaundiced, phototherapy can be used to help the body cope. The baby's eyes are covered and the body is illuminated with a light which breaks down the pigments in the body so that the baby can excrete them in its urine.

Almost all premature and low birth-weight babies will need to be kept in an incubator. This regulates the baby's temperature and enables the medical staff to give any treatment that is necessary. However, it can be very hard for the mother to relate to her baby if he or she is in an incubator, especially if surrounded by special tubes and equipment. Feeding can also be a problem. All premature babies should be given breast milk if at all possible, as this is the very best food for the baby, but the baby may be unable to suck. Some babies who are too weak to breast-feed may be able to suck from a bottle filled with expressed milk. Others may need to be fed through a tube. However, the mother of a premature baby will usually be shown how to express breast milk to provide for and nourish the baby and to establish her milk supply for when the baby is well. If a mother cannot provide breast milk, most hospitals have a milk bank available.

It was quite a business, going to the hospital all the time and expressing milk – I found it too difficult to express much at home, although I did this too. But the staff were wonderfully supportive and it made me feel as if I was really helping, was really giving him something no one else could. But it's hard, because though he's home now he's been too weak to feed from the breast and is used to the bottle, and I don't feel I can go on expressing for ever, so I don't suppose I will establish proper breast-feeding, though I'll give it a try.

Very small babies may look tiny, fragile, even ugly little creatures to begin with, which may make relating to them more difficult. The cry of a premature baby may sound more like the bleat of a lamb or mew of a kitten than the cry of a proper baby and many babies are so thin they look more like fledgling birds:

She was so tiny I couldn't believe it – she weighed only two and a half pounds. She hardly looked human at all, like a little bird that had been pushed out of the nest. Because she had breathing difficulties her little chest heaved and she made funny wheezing noises. She was surrounded with tubes and I wasn't allowed to hold her, so I felt completely unable to relate to her at all.

But despite their initial problems, the great majority of premature babies will thrive and eventually make up the time lost to them. It is important for the parents to remember, though, that their baby is really the age from the time he should have been born, not his actual birthday. One mother explains:

Since he was born three months early, it was terribly difficult explaining to people. At six months from his birth day, he was of course at the stage of a normal three-month-old baby. If I said to people, he's six months old, they would tut-tut and obviously think he was backward. So in the end I gave his age from the due date, not his birthday to casual contacts. And it was very odd celebrating his first birthday when he was just like a nine-month-old.

By the second and third birthday, of course, the difference between the baby's age and the developmental stage has narrowed and become unimportant – the baby has 'caught up'.

Stillbirth

The death of a baby is a traumatic experience and one which staff in hospitals may find it difficult to deal with. They are geared up to dealing with the joy of birth and not the tragedy of death. At the time, doctors and nurses may be taken up with dealing with the aftermath of the delivery or in trying to save a baby's life and have little time for the mother and father, leaving both in a state of uncertainty:

The delivery was ghastly and he was rushed off to special care the moment he was born. I remember they were all fussing around giving me stitches and cleaning me up, but nobody mentioned the baby. I just assumed he was dead; at first I couldn't believe it, I felt numb, then I started crying. Nobody said anything to me and my husband went off to find someone who would tell him what was going on. Then they came to take me back to the ward and I said, in tears, 'I'm not going, I'm not going to the ward to see those mothers and babies'. 'Why not? they asked. 'Because my baby's dead!' I bawled. At that there was a flurry and someone came to say he wasn't dead at all, he was in intensive care but they were sure he'd be all right and I could go back and look at him later. It was, in fact, touch and go, but they didn't say so at the time.

And if a woman is kept uninformed and uninvolved, the consequences can be quite tragic:

It was obvious that something was wrong as soon as he was born and he was taken to the special care unit. There was some confusion over what different doctors said about whether he would live or not, and I found that hard, as I didn't know whether there was hope; meanwhile I was in the normal ward with mothers and babies. I wasn't there when they disconnected the life-support system and let him die – there was no point in doing anything. If I had been more involved and helped by them I think I would have chosen to be with him and to have held him when he died.

There are probably many women who would have very similar feelings and reactions. Until very recently parents were not encouraged even to see their baby, who was whisked away as soon as it was confirmed that the baby was dead. Now, however, hospitals are increasingly aware that many parents want to see their baby and accept its death and have some time to grieve. This applies even if the baby is born with some congenital abnormality; the imaginings of someone who has given birth to an abnormal baby are likely to be much worse than the reality, and again, seeing, being with and holding the child helps parents to accept:

> They said the baby was deformed and I didn't want to see. But my husband did, and he said, really it's all right, she's quite beautiful, you can look. They had wrapped her up so that her face and arms and tiny feet showed and she was very beautiful, and her face had a peaceful expression that made me at once feel much better about her death.

A mother whose baby has died can ask not to go to the post-natal ward, but be given a room of her own or perhaps to the general gynaecological ward. Hormones can be given to suppress the milk, though they are not always given nor are they completely effective. The mother whose baby has died will have all the usual hormonal and emotional changes following a birth, but no baby; she is in a kind of limbo, neither a mother nor not a mother.

If the baby has died due to some lack of intervention or action by medical staff, parents usually take out their anger on the hospital and this can make the situation worse immediately after the baby has died: 'They should have picked up that he was in distress, I can't forgive them.' Anger is a normal part of the grieving process, and being able to blame someone can help make the situation seem more bearable for the parents in the short term. Most stillbirth or neonatal deaths, however, could not have been prevented and blaming hospitals will not bring back a baby who has died.

How the hospital staff deal with a tragedy can make an enormous difference to the experience, so if you do have any worries it can help to talk to them in advance about what you would like to happen in the event of the baby's death, even if this sounds as if you are being unnecessarily morbid:

> I told them that if the baby was dead I didn't want them to whisk her away, I would like to see and hold the baby straight away and deal with my emotions then and there. They brushed this aside and said, of course nothing will go wrong – and of course my baby was born perfectly healthy. But I felt it was important for me to say what I wanted in case the unthinkable happened, so we knew where we stood and I wouldn't be faced with half truths or well-meaning attempts to protect me from reality.

Women – and men – who have experienced the death of a baby are often told by doctors, hospital staff, relatives and friends to 'forget about the experience – you'll soon have another one'. This is very distressing for the parents who need to acknowledge the death and mourn the loss of their baby before going on to another pregnancy. Some hospitals will help the parents by encouraging them to see and hold the baby, perhaps taking a photograph which they can keep, and discussing what sort of funeral arrangements should be made. Hospitals usually arrange for a cremation or burial free of charge, but some parents find they hastily go along with such arrangements and later are distressed because they did not attend any ceremony and the baby is buried with others or in an unmarked grave.

You will also need to register the baby's birth or death – if the baby was born dead there is a special stillbirth register, and you can ask that the baby's name is recorded so that he or she can be acknowledged as your child, a real individual, and not just 'a baby'. If you feel the hospital is not paying attention to your wishes, be firm and ask for what you want; it may help you feel a lot better about the experience when you look back on it and help you in the natural process of grieving.

Bonding with your baby

Much emphasis has been placed on the importance of mothers bonding with their new baby. It is sometimes described as if 'bonding' is some mystical process which must take place in the early moments after the birth or at least within the first few days or the mother and child relationship will be in trouble. The process of bonding with a child is a very important one, but everyone is different. Some people will fall in love with their future husbands at first sight, others build a relationship slowly over the years. In the end the quality of love achieved may not have much to do with the feelings you felt at first; it is the same with a baby.

There is no doubt, though, that the conditions at the time of the birth can help the mother relate to her baby or hinder her. Hospitals have on the whole changed enormously in this respect:

My first baby, whom I had in my twenties, was born in the way it was always done; my husband wasn't there; I did what I was told. The midwife delivered the baby and I just happened to be there. The baby was taken away and bathed as soon as she was born and I was given this clean white bundle to look at. We only saw the babies at feeding time every four hours and I had to struggle to breast-feed. My husband only saw his child hours later at visiting time.

With this baby it was completely different. Not only was Peter there at the birth, he'd come along for tests and things throughout the pregnancy. It was a pleasant room with pretty wallpaper and curtains, and we could take our own things with us. The birth was fine, although I had a massive haemorrhage afterwards and the baby needed resuscitation – but as soon as all that had been seen to they left us, melted away and turned down the lights and we were left on our own with the soft lighting, pretty wallpaper and music!

Nowadays most mothers who breast-feed their baby will be allowed or encouraged to put the baby to the breast soon after the birth. The baby may be delivered straight onto the mother's tummy and in any case, both parents are likely to be able to see and hold him straight away before he is washed and weighed. Despite this kind of care, however, not all mothers feel a rush of love:

> It was a perfect birth; I saw him born, they delivered him onto my tummy, and there he was, a perfect, beautiful baby with wide open eyes; he didn't yell but looked all round him. I didn't feel a thing – in fact, at this greatest moment of my life, all I said was, 'Is that my baby?' I was completely exhausted and drained of any emo-tion. My husband held him while I was stitched up – I'm sure he bonded with him, because I could hear this long conversation going on, my husband talking to him and gazing up at his face. Then they put him to the breast, but again I didn't feel anything. It was a strange blur.
>
> Afterwards, when I was on the ward, I would look at this tiny baby next to me and think, this is it, you should be overjoyed, this is your

perfect baby. And to tell the truth, I don't think I did really love him. I mothered him, and did everything I should, felt protective and concerned, but only now he's a person and walking and starting to talk can I say that I really love him.

Nonetheless, the importance of the early time after the birth must not be underestimated. It can be important to have a time of peace and quietness together before being plunged into all the problems and worries of parenting. The time immediately after the birth provides a perfect time for this. To begin with, the baby is usually awake and alert and not yet frantic to feed. The parents can hold and talk to him and feel that he is really theirs. There need be no other distractions at this time and tasks like bathing the baby, and tidying up the mother can wait. It is a unique moment which should be exploited to the full. Some studies have shown that mothers who have been separated from their babies immediately after the birth find it more difficult to bond, and this does seem to be true of women who have had Caesarian sections or whose babies have had special care. But there are other factors as well. Women who have had infertility problems or have suffered the loss of a baby may have blocked off their emotions in case they do not get their longed-for baby; it can be more difficult to let these emotions out when the baby becomes a reality:

> I had taken a long time to conceive and also had a miscarriage. I began to think that I would never have a baby. When he was born, I think I felt that I

couldn't just switch on the love which I'd been bottling up all those years. I had to take time to get used to the fact that this was real and time to get to know him.

Some women find that being in hospital makes it more difficult for them to relate to their babies. With all the activity going on, the streams of visitors to yourself and other mothers, the comings and goings of doctors and nurses, there can seem to be little time alone to get to know your baby. Worse, your partner can only visit and when he is with you there is little privacy:

> On the fourth day I had the blues that everyone seems to have, when your milk comes in and your hormones are all upside down. I felt I couldn't cope so I went and hid in a room off the nursery to have a good cry. Then some mother came to find me and said, 'your baby's screaming its head off, what are you doing?' So I went back to feed the baby. She came with me and I know she was trying to help, she said, 'Oh, we've all had the weeps, don't worry about it.' But she kept making comments about how I was feeding the baby. I just wanted to be alone, and I wanted my husband there, especially at nights. I would lie awake at nights wanting just to cuddle him and when he did come of course all I could get was a peck on the cheek with everyone else around.

Many women feel that the time after the birth should be one for them and their families alone:

> Despite having a Caesarian I left after

six days in hospital. They said you shouldn't be leaving but I wanted the three of us to be together – I thought we'd muddle through better than here where there's all this help, yes, but it's clinical and not emotional.

> I came home after one day because I didn't want my little boy to come and see us in hospital. I didn't want him to find me stuck in a strange hospital bed and the baby in a plastic crib and unable to be ourselves. I thought he should see us all at home and get to know the baby there, to have his mother with him and not to have to go away and leave us in a strange place.

Today it is normally accepted that the father will be present at the birth of the child. This is one of the greatest changes that has taken place in the last few decades of child-bearing practice although, before hospital births became the norm, many fathers would have been present at home for their child's birth. Few hospitals make any objection to the father's presence even at difficult births like forceps deliveries or Caesarians, and the father is often involved in holding the baby after the birth. Visiting hours have also been made more flexible so that at most hospitals fathers have unlimited visiting and can get to know their child a little before they are all at home together.

A great many fathers find the whole experience of birth exciting and rewarding and say they feel closer to their children because of it. Others may also feel that they were helpless and couldn't do anything to prevent their partner's suffering which they found very up-setting. Not all men provide the help expected:

> He went green and looked terrible. I really felt for him, it made it worse for me in a way – I kept thinking I just can't yell, it'll upset him too much.

> At the worst stage in the labour I asked him how he was feeling and he said, 'I'd rather be at home in bed.' I think he just felt helpless. I felt really betrayed by him, that he could be so insensitive at that moment – but then he finds it very hard to show his feelings and he had to put on a masculine front.

> They offered me pain relief and I decided to take it, despite our plans for a natural birth. But he refused to let me take anything. He kept telling the staff, 'She doesn't mean it, she's OK.' In a way I'm pleased in retro-spect, but at the time I thought, 'What does he know about how I am feeling?

Other women feel that they could not have managed without their partners:

> He was wonderful. It helped knowing he was there and he really soothed me. When the baby was born he was so thrilled, he was beside himself. He was holding the baby as soon as they would give him to him – I wouldn't have had him miss out on that for the world.

Where the father is unable or unwilling to attend, most hospitals will allow you to have a close friend or relative as your birth partner to provide support and help. Sometimes the hospital staff seem to discourage an early discharge because they feel you will be unsupported at home. This is often not the case; many women find that they can relax and solve problems once they have sole charge of the baby and do not feel they have to get permission all the time to do what they feel most comfortable about:

> I was having problems with feeding; I had sore nipples and couldn't get the baby to latch on properly. The midwives all helped but the more advice they gave me the more confused and inadequate I felt. The atmosphere in the ward was frenetic and I was on edge all the time. I told the midwife I wanted to go home and she said, 'you're not ready yet, wait till you've got the feeding established'. I said, 'But I'll be much better at home, there won't be any interruptions'. 'Of course there will be,' she said, 'the phone will ring.' 'I'll take it off the hook,' I said. 'Then the doorbell will go.' 'Then I'll ignore it,' I said. She seemed to be looking for difficulties.

However, there has been a steady trend towards women going home from hos-pitals earlier. The once accepted, two-week stay has gone down to an average of five or six days, and many women with no problems can be discharged after 48 hours.

Breast-feeding

The majority of women leaving hospital today are breast-feeding their babies. Many hospitals now give great support and encouragement to mothers who want to breast-feed, recognizing that it is the best food for a baby and that there are emotional rewards for the nursing mother. But some women decide that they do not want to breast-feed and there is no reason why they should feel guilty about it, as there are excellent artificial baby milks now available which are made to match the mother's milk as closely as possible from the nutritional point of view. Bottle-fed babies also thrive and love is more important than the way you choose to feed, though many mothers choose to express their love through breast-feeding.

Breast-feeding is best for a baby because it is composed of exactly what the baby needs at any time. After the birth a mother produces colostrum – a yellowish fluid rich in antibodies which protects the baby from infection. It also contains protein, water and minerals in just the right proportion for the baby's first few days, and a natural laxative which helps the baby's bowels to get moving. When the milk comes in it is also perfectly balanced for the baby's needs. (Research has shown that milk produced by the mothers of premature babies is different from the normal milk and ideally suited for them.) In hot weather the milk is more watery so the baby gets enough fluid and, as the baby grows, its composition changes gradually to match this. None of this is possible with artificial baby milks.

Many hospitals send mothers home with a free tin of formula. This tends to encourage mothers to use it if the baby appears dissatisfied after one feed or if she is very tired. Do resist this temptation it takes some time to establish breast feeding and there are often initial problems, but they should sort themselves out. In giving formula you may undo some of the good you have done in choosing to breastfeed.

Starting feeding

It is important to feel comfortable and relaxed when you are breast-feeding. Get into a position which puts no strain on your back, shoulders or limbs and hold the baby comfortably, perhaps resting on a pillow so he is the right height. Use his feeding reflex to get him to feed – brush his cheek nearest the breast and he will turn his head, mouth open, to latch on.

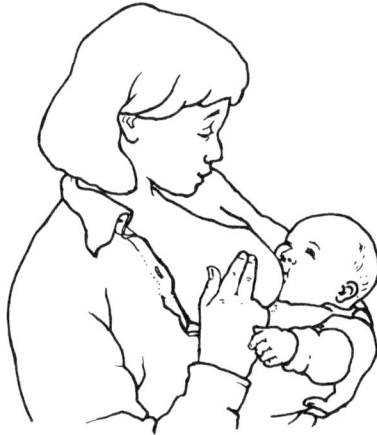

It is very important to see that the baby has the whole of the areola, the area around the nipple, in his mouth. If he has just the nipple you will soon become terribly sore and he will not be able to get the milk out. Once he is latched on properly and feeding, you should not feel any discomfort, even if your nipples are sore. If you do feel any pain, remove his mouth by slipping your little finger in to break the suction and try again.

It is usually recommended that you start off feeding for 5-6 minutes a side, building up to ten or so, to help prevent sore nipples. However, at the end of the feed the baby is likely to be sucking very gently for comfort only and if this is sending him to sleep there seems to be little point in removing him till he is satisfied.

Because breast-feeding does not come naturally to the majority of women and because it is easy to be put off by initial difficulties, many mothers need a great deal of support to establish breast-feeding. It may be particularly difficult to establish breast-feeding after a Caesarian:

The most difficult time was the first few weeks. Because I couldn't exclusively feed him I had to supplement, which was very disappointing. I did everything under the sun to try and get him to breast-feed exclusively. I had a lot of support but because of the Caesarian I had an infection and had to take antibiotics which were not compatible with breast-feeding and which I didn't question at the time, although I should have done. This all militated against breast-feeding and, of course, they put him on formula straight away in hospital – which again I would question if I had to go through it again. We got through

it, but it was a very difficult time. I think because I was older that I should have known how to cope – that somehow I shouldn't have felt so demoralized and uncoping in those first few weeks.

With other difficulties to overcome the initial experience may be unrewarding as well as discouraging. And it may take time and a lot of encouragement to get over these hurdles:

After a Caesarian I suppose I had a bad start in establishing breast-feeding and now she's six weeks old or so we have only just sorted them out. They said after a Caesar it takes longer for the milk to come in and it's difficult to hold a baby when you're feeling so sore. Also my breasts were so painful – the nipples so sore – nobody had prepared me for that. I kept thinking, 'where is this wonderful experience? Am I normal?' Finally, it was talking to a relative which helped – she said, 'yes, it is painful but it will get better'. I think in a way I had too much information and advice – I changed to the bottle as the midwife advised it and then back to the breast – I just needed someone to say, 'yes, it is awful at the beginning and I've been through it and it does get rewarding in the end'.

Many women are given the impression that they must either totally breastfeed or bottlefeed and there is no 'in between':

'I only lasted six weeks and I didn't really enjoy it. It was too demanding. The first few weeks it did take me a while to adjust to the demands. I felt as if I had done nothing but have my chest out of my sweater and with Bill away I had so much to see to. But nobody ever said to me that you could do bottle and breast. If they had I might have gone on longer. But I was rushing back to feed her and thinking, 'oh my god, I've been two and a half hours. She'll be needing another feed'. It really got me uptight and I said, 'I'm not going to do this any more', and I just stopped, which I suppose was very silly. Nobody points this two way thing out to you–that you can mix the two. You have it in your head that it's one thing or the other.'

While it may be true that it is important to breastfeed entirely for the early weeks while you are building up a good supply, the odd 'relief' bottle which a partner or childminder can give can be a great bonus and prevent a mother from giving up entirely:

I only breast-fed for six weeks. I found it too demanding – she never lasted for two hours – wanted feeding all the time. No one said you could breast *and* bottle-feed. So I just stopped and put her on a bottle which she took quite well. I didn't ask advice from the health visitor–I didn't get on with her. I'd feel all right until I saw her and then she'd upset me–that didn't help. At the baby clinic I had to wait so long I didn't bother.

Even if you are going back to work quite soon after the birth, breast-feeding for the first few weeks gives the baby the best possible start and you can continue to breast-feed morning and night if you choose.

Breast-feeding is a completely different experience to bottle-feeding and cannot be fitted into the idea of strict schedules and routines which were prevalent a generation ago. Breast-feeding mothers, who know they should feed on demand and as often as every two hours if the baby wants it, find it annoying and discouraging to hear others say, 'You can't be feeding him again, surely?' The frequent lack of understanding among older relatives and friends and even professionals means that many mothers are discouraged needlessly from breast-feeding in the early weeks. Support groups like the National Childbirth Trust (NCT) and the Laleche League can be very helpful. Most local NCT groups have a breast-feeding counsellor who can help mothers with any worries or problems.

If you do have problems, try to persevere. Apart from the physical advantages of breastfeeding for the baby, breastfeeding offers a unique bond of closeness between mother and baby once initial problems have been overcome:

I simply can't imagine not having fed my baby myself. It was the most wonderful thing that whenever I was exhausted or she was fretful we could just sit down and relax and be totally absorbed in one another. It was so easy, so natural, and made me at once feel at peace with myself and the baby . . . even at four am, it was easy just to pick her up and latch her on and sometimes I would doze back to sleep too. And it was a wonderful feeling as she grew to feel that I had done it all myself.

Table 4   Breast-feeding – common problems

Problem	Effect	What to do
Sore nipples	Especially in the early days the nipples can become very sore and painful. You may even get small blisters and sores. Very sore nipples may be caused by a fungal infection which may also affect the baby.	The hospital or midwife may recommend sprays or creams to ease this and it is important to make sure the baby is latched on properly and is not tugging or chewing on the nipple. Sunlight and fresh air help dry the nipples and soothe them.
Cracked nipples	If nipples are allowed to get too sore a crack may occur – this can be terribly painful.	You may find it helps to express from that breast for 24 hours to allow the skin to heal. Ask the midwife or doctor for advice.
Engorged breasts	This often happens when the milk comes in and before the baby gets feeding established. If the breasts are too full the baby cannot get the nipple and areola into the mouth and feed properly, so a vicious circle results.	Ask the midwife to show you how to express, and express some milk before you start feeding.
Blocked duct	You may notice a hard patch in one breast and that your breast becomes engorged behind it – this is a blocked duct. If it is not cleared it will get very painful and possibly infected.	Put the baby to the blocked breast first so that he sucks most strongly on that side. If you wait till he is very hungry this may help. Change his position at the breast and massage the lump to help it clear.

Problem	Effect	What to do
Abcess	This can result from a blocked duct which gets infected. If the breast becomes red and sore and you feel shivery or hot see your doctor at once.	Seek medical advice before continuing feeding from the infected breast.

The post-natal check

Six weeks after the birth you will return to the hospital or your GP for a check-up to ensure that your body is returning to normal after the birth. The doctor will feel your abdomen to check that the womb has returned to its normal size. Your blood pressure and weight will also be noted. You will be asked if you have had any unusual bleeding, pain or discomfort. (It is quite common for the lochia – the blood loss after the birth – to continue for more than six weeks, and some women have already had a period by this time.) Any scars from tears or episiotomies will be checked and your breasts and nipples may be examined if you have problems with breastfeeding.

You may also discuss contraception with your doctor if this has not already been arranged. Women who use a diaphragm will usually have it refitted at the post-natal check, although everything may not have returned to its normal shape and size and it may need checking again a few weeks later. An IUD can also be refitted at six weeks – it cannot usually be done immediately after the birth because there is a high chance of its being expelled if the womb is still contracting in size. If you want to take the pill, the usual combined oestrogen/progestogen pill is not suitable if you are breast-feeding as it affects the milk supply. The mini-pill or progestogen-only pill can be taken within seven days of the birth, although some mothers do not like the idea of taking any drug while breast-feeding. Many couples rely on the sheath as a temporary measure as it really is an ideal method at this time.

You will have the opportunity to raise any worries you have about your own health or that of the baby, including problems with breast-feeding. You may like to raise any worries you have about sex, especially if you have attempted intercourse and found it painful. It is very common not to have had sexual intercourse till after this post-natal stage – indeed, many women find that they need the reassurance of the post-natal check that all is well before they do so.

If you did not have a cervical smear taken earlier in pregnancy, now is a good time to have it done.

CHAPTER SIX

Afterwards

So much emphasis is put on getting pregnant, going through the nine months' preparation for childbirth and childbirth itself, that there is a tendency to forget, that in many ways, the real beginning starts after the baby is born.

Emotional and physical reactions

The first few weeks are a period of immense change and adjustment. The mother herself has been through considerable emotional and physical changes during the pregnancy. She has experienced what must be for every woman indescribable joy, pleasure and happiness – delivering, holding and nursing her baby in the first moments of his or her life. These are overwhelming emotional experiences which are totally different to anything she has ever experienced before.

But after the flood of emotion there is, quite suddenly, the reality to be faced of a new baby, dependent for his or her every need – to be fed, clothed and loved; and the realization for the parents of the enormous reponsibility they carry for the baby's welfare for many years to come. It is not surprising, then, that many women come down to earth with something of a jolt and some hit the so-called 'baby blues' a few days after the baby is born. It is a very common and perfectly normal reaction, affecting something like half of all women who have babies. Some women feel very emotional and upset and weepy for no obvious reason. Others get tense and anxious and worry that they may not be able to cope with the baby, or they may feel quite competent to cope with the baby's needs but feel very unwell and tired. Occasionally, a woman may feel a temporary loss of interest in her baby – she may even resent that she is no longer the centre of attraction:

I went through a phase, after the birth, of feeling very emotionally fragile and weepy. The slightest thing would have me in tears. I cried a lot. Along with the joy of having this baby was also an anti-climax. Suddenly people weren't looking after you any more – it was the baby who was the focus of attention. I sort of just wanted to be looked after. I remember the doctor saying 'You'll be so pleased to get out of here', and feeling, 'But I want to stay here, I don't want to go home yet.' I'm sure it is very largely to do with changes in hormones – it's such a huge change emotionally and physically to suddenly have a baby.

Women whose experience of childbirth has been disappointing in some way – because of intervention or because they were not conscious for the birth – are also more likely to go through a period of depression immediately afterwards.

For most, this period does pass quite naturally. But, for a small number of women, the 'baby blues' gets worse and becomes quite a serious depression, which does not clear. The symptoms vary widely with the individual, but usually a woman feels very sad and despondent, unable to cope with the baby, often fearful for herself and the baby. If she is having difficulty in sleeping and has little appetite, then she is likely to get more tense, irritable and exhausted. Once a vicious circle such as this sets in, it really is important that she gets medical help rather than go on suffering these distressing symptoms.

Post-natal depression can be treated successfully, although recovery may take a little while. Apart from drug treatment, most women benefit from talking about their depression rather than keeping it 'bottled up' inside. Women are often helped by talking to others who have had post-natal depression, and the Assocation for Post-Natal Illness will help those women wishing to make contact with others by putting them in touch with women who have recovered.

But depression can affect any woman who is isolated, tired and lonely at any time, so it is important to plan ahead for help and support during the early months. Looking after herself is important for the woman's welfare and that of the baby. He is dependent on her and a mother who is depressed is unlikely to be able to respond willingly or positively to her child's needs and demands.

It may be that women who have anticipated the changes in their life style and how much is involved in caring for a new baby are better prepared for this stage and less likely to go through a time of distress. Certainly being prepared would mean that women understand that it is an exhausting time, that they do need some help and they should be prepared for the first few weeks to be very much absorbed by the baby's needs:

Coming home was pretty awful because I was so exhausted and I had no one to help out at first. I had sore nipples and would have given up breast feeding if it hadn't been for my husband and his encouragement: No one tells you how painful it is. I got help for two weeks and began to feel all right again, but it was the most traumatic period of my life. I felt that I didn't know what to do. I expected it all to be intuitive, but I had absolutely no idea what the demands were. That was a shock – the realization that you were totally at the beck and call of someone suddenly. You couldn't possibly not feed them if you were tired – that was a big shock. I was a bit disappointed in the NCT. I felt that they should have led into the process of how to cope *after* the birth. I felt you were left completely alone afterwards.

Fatigue and exhaustion does seem to be one of the concerns of being an older mother and even 'experienced' mothers may find themselves getting very tired:

> My first was a very sweet-natured baby, but Richard was a difficult baby. He was colicky for the first few months. You know babies are different but you assume that you are going to have another one like the one before and he just screamed solidly for the first three months. I think at one point I did think that my age might have something to do with it and that I was older and not coping so well and that he sensed it and I was much tireder. I was child-minding, but then I could have had two toddlers of my own at home . . . . I thought maybe because I was tired he was sensing it and being more irritable. But it was a harder first year than it was with the first one.

In fact this woman had moved house just before her son was born, and with so much to do she herself admitted that it was not surprising that she felt so tired: 'I needed to go and sort out the kids' toys or unpack a tea chest and I just couldn't and that frustrated me as well.'

Clearly major practical upheavals such as moving house are best avoided at this time. But perhaps also some women have unrealistic expectations of how they are likely to feel at the end of a day looking after babies and small children. Women who simply accept that they are going through a tiring period in their lives and make the necessary adjustments seem to cope well:

> 'I'm definitely whacked by the end of the day and I need to go to bed reasonably early because Karen is up early in the morning. I usually go about ten. He (my husband) is away from time to time and I'm off to bed like a shot – 9 o'clock if I can.'

The fact is that caring for babies and small children is physically hard work. But it may be that being tired is more to do with life style and one of the ways to avoid fatigue is for women to keep fit, eat a healthy diet and generally look after themselves – as well as their families:

> A lot of people say it's more tiring having children when you're older. I can't really compare. Certainly I'm in much better physical shape than I was a few years ago – I don't smoke now and I exercise. I weigh less and I have lots of energy. So that to me is not an issue. Certainly you get tired when you go for years without a child sleeping through the night as we did with Matthew. But I don't think I was any more tired than I would have been if I was younger.

Keeping fit and healthy these days does not mean staying slim through starvation. If you find the type of exercise you enjoy, it will improve your general health, keep you in good shape, help you to relax mind and body and generally make you feel better. Many women find that increasing the amount of regular exercise they take helps to overcome feelings of lethargy and tension. Any form of aerobic exercise – jogging, swimming or keep-fit type exercises – will improve fitness and stamina. You can do these on your own or make them part of an enjoyable social outing by joining a class.

In general, a good healthy diet is one that contains plenty of fresh fruit and vegetables, fish, chicken and fibre (wholemeal bread, pasta and potatoes). Foods to cut down are red meats, fats, sugar, refined and processed foods, as well as alcohol, tea and coffee. If your eating pattern involves missing out on breakfast, a very light lunch and eating a large meal in the evening, try changing the balance and starting the day with a good nutritious breakfast to give you energy. If you are breast-feeding your baby, you will need to keep up your calorie intake and try to have a nourishing snack or drink at the baby's feeding times to maintain your energy.

Support

Traditionally, a woman would have looked first to her own mother or her partner's mother for help and support in the early months of being on her own with her baby. But parents who have their first child over 30 often have less support from their own families because they may have lost one or both parents. If parents are getting elderly and in failing health they may be in need of a lot of care themselves and may simply not be able to help out at this time.

In some cases women who are older, and have clear ideas about how they want to bring up their child, prefer to do it in their own way without too much help from mothers or mothers-in-law:

My mother would have just been a nuisance telling me I was doing things all wrong. She had very different ideas. She couldn't understand why Julia was always up in the evenings wanting to be fed. She thought babies should be tucked up in bed. She had long since forgotten. It is a disadvantage of having babies late – your mother is even further removed from it all.

But the value of support from some source should not be underestimated: 'With my own mother dead, I desperately needed a friend who was a mum herself. Nothing prepares you for it – sleepless nights – I never knew how long they went on for, it seemed like months and months.'

This is a time to search out and rely on good friends whom you can talk to and who have some experience of babies in common with you. Much of the normal everyday exchange of what may seem like unimportant chat is essential for new mothers. Babies and children so often behave in ways which seem antisocial, or appear to be progressing more slowly than they should, that it is very easy for a mother to feel inadequate. And with so many so-called 'experts' on child care, she needs to be reminded occasionally that the real expert on her child is the mother herself. Getting feedback and reassurance from others helps a lot of women to build up their own self-confidence – that they may not be perfect but they are doing a good job: 'I relied on friends to talk to and say, "Simon's been doing something ghastly", and who would say, "Oh, that's nothing, my older one did the same thing for years and years, but he grew out of it," – that sort of thing. I find friends very useful that way.'

If you are a single mother, it is even more important to have family and friends to rely on. Some mothers find they have to call on everyone close to them for support, especially in the early weeks:

> I had a difficult labour, and was exhausted. When I went home I was ruthless. I rang all my friends and organized a rota for them to come so I wasn't actually on my own in the house for a month after the birth.

Lack of self-confidence may be particularly hard for women who have had a career, been good at their job and felt they have achieved certain things:

> Suddenly I'm a beginner. I don't know the answers and that really threw me. It was so frightening. Normally you would think, 'Never mind, hang on, go and read a book.' But there are no books, no one can tell you. The more you ask the more conflicting it gets. You just have to sit and learn and stick it out.

Older parents may run the risk of being more isolated than younger parents if they move in circles where their friends do not have babies and small children. If friends are not so readily accessible, many women get the same sort of support from meeting with other mothers at mother-and-toddler groups or National Childbirth Trust post-natal groups. In this case, the mother found invaluable help with a breast-feeding problem: 'I was happy about the breast-feeding because I got a lot of support from the NCT – there was always someone in the group having similar problems to you so you didn't feel isolated.'

Women with young babies are particularly vulnerable to the dangers of being isolated and lonely, more so because the provision for mothers with babies under one year is still very patchy. In the last few years, however, there has been a considerable increase in the number of informal mother-and-toddler groups and those like the NCT.

Most mother-and-toddler groups are run by parents themselves or through organizations like NCT, the Pre-school Playgroup association and Meet-A-Mum (MAMA). These organizations will act as contact points for parents who want to get together to form a group. Their main aim is to provide a pleasant meeting place for parents (usually mothers), as well as a safe play area, with toys and equipment, for the babies and toddlers. The parents are responsible for their own children, but are also able to make friends with people of similar interests and discuss issues about child-rearing which concern them. In the absence of the old-style, extended family, these groups do fill a gap and provide a much needed means of valuable support for parents who might otherwise be on their own.

Similar groups are also run at local health clinics, surgeries or in community centres. They are mostly run informally, again offering women a chance to meet and talk. In some cases there are opportunities to follow Open University courses on parenting and these are more formal and structured.

Health visitors, who are experts in child care, may organize groups of this sort.

The health visitor is one of the key people for any new mother to maintain contact with. She is a valuable source of good advice and support. Not only is she knowledgeable about child health and development, but she usually knows the local scene very well and can put women in touch with local groups and activities.

Older children

Older mothers with older children (or stepmothers of older children) have to think about how a baby is likely to affect their lives, and how the needs of a baby, school-age or teenage children can be met at the same time. Parents having a 'second family' may also fear jealousy on the part of older siblings or half-siblings.

Older children may not be so dependent but they, as well as teenage children, still need a great deal of time and patience – perhaps more so if they feel even slightly threatened by the imminent arrival of a new member of the family. Children in these situations react differently and not always as expected:

> I thought they would be terribly embarrased about the whole thing or jealous, but they were thrilled.'

> Jane was very helpful. She would come in from college at night and say, 'Don't worry, I'll make the tea,' if I was tired. We never had any problems. When I hear about all the traumas other people went through with their teenage children – I've been pretty lucky.

But young people have their own preoccupations at this time and while they may enjoy the new baby, they may resent being expected to be on hand as baby-sitters. They may be going through the difficult process of 'spreading their wings' in readiness for leaving the comfort and security of home, and it may require no small effort for a couple with a new baby to make sure relationships with their older children are reinforced at this time:

> Andrew gets in from school at four and we usually sit down and have a cup of tea, and just chat about the day – and I always try and make sure that we all sit down to eat together in the evening – although more and more these days he is rushing off somewhere.

In some cases, having a baby and a teenager in a house causes great problems. Young people want to play their music, have friends in and are often generally noisy, just at a time when parents of a young baby may be exhausted and in need of peace and quiet. Parents in situations like these insist that being patient, more understanding and tolerant is far more likely to create a 'give and take' situation which works for everyone. It is when life is made to revolve entirely around the baby that difficulties arise, although it is often the baby which provides the focus for expressing the bonds which tie the whole family:

I always felt rather awkward with my stepchildren till Richard arrived. They both made a great fuss of him and that made us closer. I could never kiss my six-foot, 16-year-old stepson to show him physical affection, but now when he comes I can say to Richard, 'Give Mark a kiss,' and he does it for me.

Older children can help of course and make life easier in practical ways, but the constant adjusting to the enquiring mind of a lively teenager and a toddler learning to talk may take some getting used to:

There are all the emotional tensions and strains. I think probably this big gap is quite difficult in a way even though I can imagine it would be very difficult to have three close together. But I find myself very much switching around – talking to a 12-year-old wanting to know about this, discussing some book that he has read and wanting to do his homework. Then teaching the little one colours and jigsaws. You have to do that all very quickly. That changing I find quite difficult. But then other people say,

well it must be quite easy with an older one, and it is in many ways – Andrew can run and get nappies, watch him in the bath if I have to answer the phone.

In practice what most women find is that there are advantages and disadvantages whatever their situation, that there is never a 'best stage' at which to have the next child. It does seem, however, that children willingly adapt to a new member of the family at any age, despite initial jealousies or problems:

We were worried about how six-year-old Laura would adjust to having a new half-sister, having been 'the baby' for so long and very spoiled in many ways. But she's shown no jealousy and is good at entertaining Sarah and looking after her. The other day Sarah tore up a painting Laura had done and I asked her if she thought Sarah a terrible nuisance. 'Well, sometimes,' she said, 'but, on the whole I would rather have a little sister than not.'

Going back to work

Making the decision

For many older mothers a major issue is whether to return to work. The considerations in terms of giving up a career or job or the opportunity of a career, the financial aspects, getting out of the house and being with other adults, the losses and the rewards all have to be weighed up against each other. Some women will want to return to work, others may settle for part-time work and there will be those who decide it is important to be at home.

In many cases, a woman may not be sure about what to do until after the baby is born:

It was only after I had the baby that I wanted to be home. I did keep the option open of going back to work, but Susie turned out to be such a demanding baby and I didn't like to leave her with a child-minder. It was taking me all my time to cope, it would not have been fair to leave her with a child-minder. I would like to get back into teaching now, but it's hard to get back.

I wouldn't leave Catherine. I really don't want to work although I didn't make that decision until after she was born. I think I made that decision in the States where they are much more family minded. People would say to me, 'What a lovely baby - my, aren't you lucky!' and I would think, 'Me! Lucky?' And it just slowly changed. Just being with her every day just slowly changed it. I'm quite happy and content at home.

That is not to say that being at home does not have its drawbacks. Housework can be a drudge and daily routines with small children can be boring. What matters is that, all in all, these women are content with what they have chosen:

There are times when every day is the same. I always think in the long term - no one else can bring up your child as well as you can. You look at friends and how they have brought up their children. There are always things you will criticize. But I'm not saying that people shouldn't go out to work - if it suits them.

Some women feel quite positively that they would be unable to do a job outside the home properly:

I would probably like to work in a few years. But I couldn't go back to teaching just yet. Teaching is very tiring and demanding. If I did I would feel that I wasn't doing either job properly. There's not enough time in the day and the children would be given what's left and the food flung in front of them. But that's not to say I want to stay home for good.

And women who have had quite demanding jobs are sometimes happy to settle for more mundane part-time work, if they can get it, which does not involve a major commitment.

What I would really like is a not very high-powered job two or three mornings a week, but not enough to intrude on the family - I would be quite happy to pack shelves in a supermarket. I think when children start school they need to be encouraged to give them a wide range of interests and activities to develop confidence in something which they can do.

Women who work

For many women there may be little choice but to return to work for purely economic reasons - many women work simply because they have to. But there are probably many couples or single women for whom a higher income may be a pressing factor, or it may be that they would find it very difficult to adjust to a lower level of income: 'We were used to having two salaries and I suppose it would have meant having to cut down quite significantly if I had given up my job - I don't know how we would have managed. In the end we just decided it would be better if I kept on my job.'

Single women may feel very strongly that they want to provide for their child and there are plenty of cases where women do this to the point of working for no more than they would receive in supplementary benefit. Having a feeling of security is what matters: 'If I was in a different situation, either living with someone or married, then things might be different. I do miss him but I know that the woman who looks after him is very good with him – and he's always pleased to see me. I feel that this is the right decision for me.'

The social aspects too are often very important – getting out and meeting people. For some women the boredom and depression of being at home all day with only a small child for company may simply not be alleviated by the range of social activities available to them – the mother-and-toddler groups and play-groups – and for them working may provide the answer.

While some women who have worked for a long time before having a baby may feel relief to be able to take on the role of full-time mother, others may feel guilty – they need to feel useful and have a sense of purpose which they may not get from being at home all day:

I know I have to work for my own development as a person and for my sanity. I'm not very patient with small children – I like them when they get to school age best. But it's not easy to tear this clinging toddler from your skirt when you leave and it's very hard if they're ill and you have to leave them with the nanny. I try not to feel guilt – I think that's destructive. But it's hard when you're being pulled in two directions – your obligation to your employer and colleagues and commitment to work, and your commitment to and love for your children.

Clearly there is more than one side to the question of working and it can be a dilemma to which there is no easy solution. Many women will have had successful careers, and for them it may be very hard to give up working. Their dilemma may never really go away:

I expected when I had children everything would become absolutely clear and I wouldn't want to work and I would be able to devote myself entirely to the children. In a way I envy anyone who feels like this but I don't, and in a way that complicates things. I miss the children dreadfully when I'm away and I get these dreadful irrational fears that something terrible has happened. But the children are very precious – I think I am terribly lucky to have two in my late thirties/early forties.

Women clearly do find their careers very satisfying and want to combine having children with their jobs, even though this does mean tremendous demands on their time and energy: 'It is hectic and it sometimes seems that life is all go – dashing to pick up kids, shopping, work – but I really love my job and I do get a lot out of it, I really couldn't think of giving it up.'

But job satisfaction itself is only one factor. For some couples, part of the recipe for the success of a marriage and family life lies in the woman having some independence and a life outside the home, where she meets other adults. Often there are a whole lot of considerations: 'Having worked for so long now, it's desperately important to me, but I try and arrange things around so that I can do both. We don't have a social home life. My husband works very long hours, so I go out to work for social reasons as well.'

One solution which many women see as an ideal compromise is part-time work, although there are fewer opportunities for part-time work in many areas where employment opportunities generally have been contracting. If a good nursery can be found, the child benefits by being in a stimulating environment. Women who do not have a lot of contact with other mothers with young babies or small children may see playgroups or nurseries as providing this function, while also giving them the chance to work some of the time:

> There are very few children round here and I think it's good for her to be in a nursery with other children. I have a part-time job in the local shop. I feel that she needs to learn to get on with other children her age and there is a lot for them to do in a nursery – it teaches them things to do.

> I'm looking forward to going back to work – it will only be part-time to begin with after Christmas when she starts nursery school – but it will be getting out of the house and meeting people. I do get a bit depressed and lonely at home.

But part-time working can also have its drawbacks for some women:

> In many ways part-time workers have it worse. The full-time working mothers have everything organized and done for them – housework, laundry, household repairs, child care and often baby-sitting. They come home to bath the kids and put them to bed. I work three days a week and on the other two I'm cleaning the house, doing the shopping, cooking the meals for the rest of the week, and taking Tom to mother and toddler groups and I'm always exhausted. Nothing is ever done, the house is a mess and we're not even that much better off.

The financial equation can be a very difficult one. Some women find that they pay out almost what they earn: 'After tax, national insurance and fares, I was bringing home about £300 a month. When I had one child £120 went on child-minding and now that I have two and can't share a nanny any longer, that's doubled. So in fact I'm working for £60 a month – that's just not worth it.'

Other women work freelance from home and find this ideal as they can fit in work around their child's needs. However, it too has problems: 'I found I'd be talking to clients while Emily was whining and yelling in my ear. Once I sat and watched her destroy one of my valuable books because I was in the middle of an important phone conversation and it was keeping her quiet.'

Work outside the home is clearly one of the needs of some women. It is very much a matter of personal choice and circumstances. Added to that most women, whatever their age when they have children, know that being completely involved in children does not last for ever. Women who see themselves as committed to this role mostly see the period spanning five or six years. After that, starting school is the beginning of the gradual process of independence:

> At the moment I'm not working, but Ben is six now and when Mark starts school I think I will look for a job. They will be mostly off my hands then and I would get very bored being in the house on my own all day. And anyway, I have the rest of my life to live. Children aren't around you for ever.

So working outside the home – either holding down a job while their children are small or returning to work after two or three years, or when their child has started school – is the reality of life for very many women. The practicalities of juggling home and job often involve a hectic life style and require some organizing if everyone is to benefit from it.

The main consideration and perhaps that which causes most concern is knowing that your child feels secure and is well looked after and happy. There are obviously many children with working mothers who do not suffer in any way. Clearly, the best way to ensure this is by knowing that you are leaving him or her in good hands.

Child care

If you are going back to work, whether full time or part time, the most important thing will be that you are satisfied with the arrangements you have made for the care of your child while you are working. There are several possibilities and it is worth spending some time looking at the alternatives, talking to other working mothers and seeing how they deal with the arrangements and the problems they have had to face.

It is worth saying at the outset that there is no evidence that small babies or children suffer through being looked after part of the time by other caring people than the parents. Indeed, being cared for sometimes by relatives such as older children and grandparents or by friends and neighbours as well as by nannies or child-minders may help the child realize that there are other sources of fun, warmth and stimulation than the mother and father and that it is quite safe to be left with them, and enjoyable too. In many cultures children are cared for by an extended family and friends and indeed, it may be unnatural for children to be only in the company of one person all the time and to depend only on that person.

At the same time, children do need security, stability and a routine and they need high standards of physical and emotional care. Leaving a child in the charge of a rapidly changing series of uncaring child-minders, nannies and baby-sitters or where there is no routine is bound to be unsettling and disturbing for a small child. It is very important that you look carefully into the arrangements you have made for your child so that you are satisfied that he or she is getting the right kind of care.

Working mothers sometimes worry that their children will become too attached to their nannies or child-minders and will not be close enough to them. However, studies have shown that even when children spend more time with other carers than with their parents, such as on a kibbutz, they still form stronger ties with their parents.

As long as parents provide the right kind of love, care and attention, there is no danger that a child will become more attached to a nanny or child-minder than to the parents. After all, for the vast majority of children of working parents, it is the mother and father who are there when they wake, go to them in the night, nurse them when they are ill, bath them and put them to bed, take them on holidays and outings and spend the weekends together. The old-fashioned nanny who stayed with the family for years or even generations and brought the children up is a thing of the past. Nannies and child-minders change, but the parents are always there.

Alternative forms of care

The four main options today for working mothers are: creches and private nurseries; day nurseries run by local authorities; child-minders (usually registered with the local council); and daily or live-in nannies.

Creches and private nurseries

Very few employers at the present time run creches or provide nursery places for their staff's children. Where there is a creche at work, this can be the ideal solution: 'It was wonderful. I knew he was right there if he needed me. I used to go down in my lunch-hour to breast-feed till he was a year old and he seemed to enjoy the company of the other children and playing with toys we just couldn't afford to have at home.'

Private nurseries are very few and also tend to be very expensive, so will not be an option for the majority of working mothers.

Local authority day nurseries

These services exist to provide full-time care for the children of full-time working mothers, and details can be obtained from the social services department of the local authority.

Because there are so few places, most will be given to the children of single parents and families with other problems. If you are offered a place, it is worth looking carefully at the facilities provided before you accept it to make sure you are happy with them, and it helps to introduce the child gradually, as the atmosphere and routine of a day nursery is very different from home.

Child-minders

A child-minder is a person who takes another child or children into her own home and cares for them for a wage. Child-minders should be registered with the local social services department – this means that the child-minder will be checked to make sure she has no record of ill-treatment of children or has not had children taken into care; that she has no police record; that her health is good and that her premises are safe. Limits are also put on how many children she can have in her care at one time and a social worker can pay a visit to check that all is as it should be.

Some child-minders do not register and it may be perfectly possible to find an unregistered child-minder who is perfect in every way, but simply does not want to become involved with authority or bureaucracy. It will be your responsibility to assess this yourself, but clearly there are advantages all round in the child-minder being registered, and you can try to persuade her to do so if she hasn't already informed the council that she is caring for your child.

One of the main advantages of using a child-minder is that such people usually have lived in the area for some years and are unlikely to move away, so are likely to provide a long-term solution to your child's care. If she does not have too many children to care for, your child will be in a family atmosphere and it will be rather like spending time with a family friend or aunt.

The disadvantages may be that the child-minder does not give the child as much attention as you would like or involve him in any educational activities. The child-minder may be tied to the house, so that your child cannot go out but spends all his time within four small walls.

Nannies
Live-in nannies are often the ideal arrangement for a working family. The nanny is in the house so that you can see for yourself how she relates to the child, and she is on hand to baby-sit for an agreed number of evenings and can also sometimes help out at the weekends. The child will be in a familiar home environment and it is as if you are simply extending your family by one member. However, you do need a large house which gives both you and the nanny privacy and nannies tend to be young, recently qualified girls who are ready to move on within a short space of time. Sometimes nannies come from a long way away and rapidly become homesick, others form new relationships and decide they want to live out rather than in. Most nannies will have meals with you or at least provided by you.

You can find nannies by advertising in certain publications – *The Lady* is the main one, through local papers or by approaching one of many nanny agencies. Agencies, however, can be expensive, although they will usually guarantee to replace someone who lets you down without leaving you in the lurch.

You can also employ a nanny, on a daily basis, who comes into your home for the hours you require. Many parents find that the best solution is to share such a nanny with someone in a similar situation so that the cost is split, and this arrangement also provides a playmate for your child. Sharing a nanny is also a very good idea for those who work part-time. You may meet other mothers wanting to share a nanny locally or through mother-and-toddler groups or organizations like the NCT, who sometimes have a nanny-sharing register. Some agencies offer a nanny-sharing scheme.

If you have advertised for a nanny, or have asked for someone to be recommended by an agency, you will want to interview each applicant. It is worth giving some thought to this. Fix a time when you will be able to give the interview time and attention, when your child is likely to be awake and perhaps when your husband or partner can meet her too.

If you are sharing a nanny, it will help if you are both there. Probably the most important thing will be your intuitive response to the nanny, whether you warm to her or not, feel at ease and how the child or children react to her. However, you can also help yourself by writing down key questions that you want to ask. These can be concerned with particular ways you would like the child to be handled and the nanny's view on various aspects of child-rearing. You can also explain the child's routine, likes and dislikes, and specify anything you would particularly like the nanny to do or not to do.

Many nannies will be qualified and have the Nursery Nursing Education Board diploma (NNEB), which means that the nanny has done a two-year course involving theoretical and practical elements of child-rearing. Not all nannies will be qualified, however; some may be mothers themselves, while others may have gained experience through nannying. You should always ask to see past references and follow these up; it will help to give you an idea of the nanny's reliability and personality.

Most nannies, especially qualified ones, will limit their tasks only to looking after children; they will not take kindly to being asked to do housework, shopping or other tasks on a regular basis. If there are things you would like done, you can always ask; the nanny may be prepared to do a little housework for a little more money, but remember this may mean she has less time to give to the child or children.

You will soon know whether the child is thriving or not under the new arrangements, and you will quickly notice if there is anything wrong with his physical care or emotional state. However, many mothers find that there are small problems or differences of opinion with their nannies or child-minders which act as a constant niggling worry:

We had brought Emma up on a no-sugar, no-additives diet and she had gone straight from breast to her teacher-beaker. I provided the food for Diane to give her, but when I got home I found crisp and biscuit wrappers in the bin and Emma started demanding 'biccies' all the time. I told Diane to give her fruit or cheese instead but it didn't seem to sink in, and I was so happy with her in every other way I didn't like to make a big fuss. Then I found she had started drinking from the other little girl, Flora's, bottle. She started asking for a bottle and that really annoyed me as she'd never had one before!

She doesn't take them out very much and I think he gets bored, because he runs riot when he gets home, running round the garden yelling his head off. He's not like that when he's here with me.

She has a friend who's a nanny in the area and she's always taking the two of them round there to play with the other three, or sometimes the other kids come here. Once I came home early and there were five children all rampaging around my living room while the two nannies were drinking tea in the kitchen. She's a very warm and caring person, though, and Sam is very fond of her, so I don't like to say anything.

Other mothers find that the nanny or child-minder adds another dimension to the child's life:

She takes them to feed the ducks in the park and to the toddler's playground. She thinks up all sorts of things for them to do – sticking bits of straw and coloured paper to sheets of paper and making dough with flour and water. When I come home I find

he's got new words and new skills – she teaches him a lot.

Jane really took the initiative with potty training and it worked wonderfully. She had done it so many times she was very cool about it, while I got in a flap and ended up with puddles all over the floor.

Finding suitable child-care arrangements is an ongoing worry for the working mother for many years; even when the child starts school, there are the school holidays to cater for and arrangements to be made when the child is ill. Having both children and a job usually means that you must have a reasonably understanding relationship with your employer, that you must be prepared to sacrifice some paid leave for caring for a sick child or stepping in when the nanny or child-minder is ill, and that your partner is prepared to make some of these sacrifices too. Otherwise, the situation may become unworkable.

Weaning to go back to work

Many working mothers worry about having to wean their babies from the breast in time to go back to work. But if you think ahead and prepare, there is no reason to stop breast-feeding or to choose bottle-feeding early on because you know you are going back to work.

If you want to go back to work before your baby is old enough to be taking enough solid food to meet his needs, it will help if you get him used to taking a bottle on a fairly regular basis – perhaps

3-4 times a week – once your milk supply is well established. The baby who is used to the breast may protest at being given a bottle:

Sam would never drink from a bottle. He screamed with rage even at the sight of one. I went out leaving him with my mother a fortnight before going back to work and he went hungry rather than have a bottle. My mother had a terrible time! In the end

I had to go home every lunchtime for the first fortnight till we persuaded him to drink from a teacher-beaker.

You can express your own milk or use a formula. Most mothers find that they can give their babies several bottles a week without any danger to breast-feeding:

> With my first child I expressed milk when necessary – I think breast-feeding with the first child is an incredible link which you feel very intense about. With Alice I put her on the odd bottle of formula from four months because it would make life so much easier. It didn't affect breast-feeding at all.

Very occasionally a baby given a frequent bottle will decide he or she prefers this and reject the breast, but this is very rare and often happens when the baby is ready for at least partial weaning anyway. Mothers who are determined not to give formula, or who return to work when their baby is very small, can usually express enough milk, although a breast pump may be necessary:

> I went back to work when Daniel was three months old. I hired a mechanical breast pump from the NCT as I didn't have much success with the little hand pumps, and I found I could easily express enough after the morning feed and at weekends and my days off to make up the bottles I needed while I was at work. Of course it isn't really very 'natural' – mechanical pump and deep freezer are necessities – but I enjoyed the feeling that I was doing it all myself.

There is no reason why working mothers should not continue to breast-feed their babies, while they are at home, for as long as they like. For many mothers a return to work at the end of the statutory 29-week period means that dropping daytime feeds falls into the weaning pattern they are pursuing anyway:

> By six or seven months he was having solids for breakfast, lunch and tea with breast milk early morning and night and in-between when he seemed hungry or needed comfort. He drank very well from a trainer cup. So dropping daytime breast-feeding was no problem. If I wasn't there he didn't seem to miss them.

Planning to be a working mother

It has now become much easier to combine motherhood and work because of the legislation on maternity leave and pay which gives mothers the right to return to their jobs after having a baby. There are also allowances payable to mothers who have worked and other benefits available for mothers who, perhaps because they are single or have partners who are unemployed, are suffering from financial hardship.

Maternity leave and pay

If you work for an employer who has a staff of more than five, you have the right to take maternity leave from eleven weeks before your baby is due up to 29 weeks after the birth, and return to your previous job, provided that you have been working for that employer for at least two years by the eleventh week before your baby is due. Your employer also has to pay you for six of these weeks, at 90 per cent of your basic pay. Your employer pays tax and national insurance contributions on this and can claim back the cost of your maternity pay from the government.

In order to claim maternity leave and pay, you must write to your employer at least three weeks before you intend to stop working, stating that you are leaving to have a baby, that you intend to come back to your job, and you also have to write and tell your employer the date you intend to return to work at least three weeks in advance of that date. In practice, of course, you are likely to discuss all this with your employer much earlier and will probably be involved in the appointment of a temporary re-placement who will be doing your job while you are away.

Many employers have in fact im-proved on this statutory minimum, and enable women who have worked for only a year before leaving to have a baby to take maternity leave, or enable them to take more than the 29 weeks after the birth, or provide more maternity pay. Other women may be able to negotiate a phased return to work, and some employers seek to provide part-time work for mothers who would like this when they return, perhaps through job sharing or job splitting arrangements. Other employers are less sympathetic; it is not unheard of for women to be passed over for promotion because they have taken maternity leave.

All pregnant women are allowed time off work for antenatal care, and some employers may give paid time off work to attend parent-craft classes. It may help if you have a letter from your doctor or midwife saying that such classes are an essential part of your antenatal care.

Some employers give paternity leave, perhaps for as long as a week or two to be taken within a fixed time either side of the birth, although this is not compulsory. Other employers will give compassionate leave to fathers when a baby is born, especially if he can get a letter from the doctor or midwife saying that it is essential that there is someone else at home to look after the new mother when she leaves hospital.

Because you will inevitably be going without pay for part of the time you are not working, it is important to find out what benefits you are entitled to claim for before and after the baby is born. Working mothers will usually be entitled to claim the statutory maternity pay or the maternity allowance, which is paid weekly, usually for 18 weeks.

Women who have worked for their employers for at least 6 months without a break by the end of the 15th week before the baby is due and have earned enough in the last eight weeks to pay Na-tional Insurance contributions qualify for statutory maternity pay at the lower rate; if they have worked for two years full time or five years part time they qualify for a higher rate for the first six weeks, equal to 90 per cent of normal pay.

Lump sums can be paid to people receiving supplementary benefit or housing benefit supplement to help them with extra expenses like maternity clothes. All mothers can claim child benefit, which is a weekly payment of £7.25 for each child. In addition, you are entitled to free NHS dental care and free prescriptions while you are pregnant and until your baby is a year old.

You may qualify, especially if you are a single parent, for other benefits such as single-parent benefit, family-income supplement and free milk and vitamins. Further information on this and other benefits, is available from the Social Security office or Citizens' Advice Bureau.

Being a full-time mother

Working outside the home has become very much the norm for a whole generation of women, with and without families. Many women who have children later in life opt for full-time domesticity – for a period, at least. Some find themselves reassessing domestic life. It may be sheer relief from what in reality was a boring and monotonous job. It may come as a great surprise to find that there is more to being a full-time mother than they thought.

Certainly most women do feel that the majority of people are dismissive of women who are 'just housewives' and there is a great deal of resentment about the way in which society fails to acknowledge how important and worthwhile a role it is:

I feel cross about the way it is denigrated. People are always saying, 'When are you going back to work?' I wouldn't consider working, although I have a lot of trouble holding up this line of argument in front of other people. But I think you have children at home for five or six years; across a few children, maybe eight or nine years. I think what I'm doing is important.

To some extent changing attitudes or different attitudes are probably largely to do with the individual and what she feels is right at any point in her life:

When I was with Susan I would have said, 'No, I want to go out to work.' Now I say, 'What's five or six years of your life to give to them while they are small?' But that's an older person speaking. Twenty years ago it was wrong for me to be in the house all the time with a child – I couldn't cope then. It was my mother who bailed me out time and time again. Whereas now, what's five or six years out of your life? It's nothing.

Many feel that it is women themselves who have contributed to the present situation, while also acknowledging that there is often a real dilemma for women:

I think it is so much more difficult now with the pressure of jobs. Two women I know had fantastic jobs but they would have had no chance of getting them back later. But with so many of them it's a case of, 'Well, it's my right to work and it's fulfilling.'

Tom has women working there who don't need the money. They say they are there to keep their minds active and that they, as people, have needs as well. To be honest, being a social worker is not the most stimulating of jobs, although it isn't trendy to say that. I think they are talking a lot of nonsense when they say they need to keep their minds stimulated. It can be much more stimulating at home.

Perhaps the 'glamour' and appeal of the career woman, so well projected by magazines and the media, is more an illusion than a reality. A long, hard look at a working woman's life may show that it is not necessarily all it's cracked up to be:

> Don't tell me that even in the most exciting jobs, there is no drudgery. I used to look after the child of a woman who was a lecturer at the university and so unspoken between us was the fact that I was doing the drudgery work and she was the stimulated alive one out in the world. It was absolutely the opposite. She wasn't interesting. I read more than she did. Her life was drudgery – getting up at the crack of dawn, waking up this child that ought to have been sleeping – hers was the drudgery. My life was so much freer. I saw more people, spoke to more people.

And the cost in terms of losing out on their children, which some women may not even be aware of, is seen as a high price to pay:

> The really sad thing was that she was also missing out on a great experience. She had a lovely child. That was the biggest thing. She was just

missing that and she just didn't know it – she just didn't spend enough time with the child to know it.

> They can have their weekends and evenings but that experience bears no relationship to having them seven days a week. If you don't know the bad bits, you don't know the good bits. If you don't know that it is absolute hell and fraught sometimes, I don't think you have brought them up. Of course they're thrilled to have them in the evenings and at weekends, but that's not what it's about.

That doesn't mean to say that being at home all day with small children is not without its drawbacks – and few women would pretend that there isn't hard work, boredom and some drudgery involved. One aspect of looking after small children is the sheer physical effort required. One woman pointed out what this could entail for her, living in a flat:

> People don't realize how physically hard work children are, even though here you are getting in and out of cars, not struggling with buses. First you have to take the pram down, then the toddler, then the baby, then repeat the whole process – sometimes just for a pint of milk! When Ben is coming home from school for lunch I can be doing that four times a day!

But many women admit that the real chores are the housework – it is boring when it is a never-ending round of cleaning, that not getting out gives them 'cabin fever', that they can be lonely from time to time and that they do get very 'fed-up':

I can't bear monotony or spending the whole day in the house. It doesn't have to be anything exciting – going to the mother-and-toddler group or going into town and getting even a pair of school socks. But if I've achieved nothing I hate it – the sameness of every day. I like to see friends most days – even if it's only at the school gates.

The thing I really hate about staying at home is the housework. There is no way I can have help in the house and that to me really is the worst bit of the whole deal.

There are many older mothers who simply give up jobs and careers because they feel very strongly about the importance of a mother being with a child. There are many women who admit quite happily that they have no desire to return to work and that they are very content being at home:

> I don't want to work while the children are small. I got so much satisfaction from when Karen was small. Whatever your showed her or talked to her about, it came back to you in other situations. It really was very satisfying. I do enjoy them while they are small.

Being at home, seeing the child grow and develop – first words and first steps – are all important. Equally important to many women is to know that they are responsible for those milestones:

> I personally would find it very hard if I wasn't seeing the things Matthew does for the first time . . . if I felt that a lot of his behaviour was to do with the way someone else was raising him, if I felt that most hours of the day he was relating to someone else and not to me. I would find that very difficult.

A woman who has waited a long time to have her first baby, because of infertility problems or for other reasons, may feel particularly strongly about bringing up her child:

> You want to give as much as you can to your child, particularly if you're older and you feel that you may not have any more children, and it may be your only chance at motherhood and you want to do the best you can for your child.

Sarah says simply that she is content to accept her role as full-time housewife and mother:

> . . . unless you have a reversal of roles where your husband is at home and you're going out to work – I think I would have liked something like that when I was younger. But I've no plans for going back to work. You do have the biggest share of the child in the first few years of its life and if you can accept that, you're OK.

Adapting, the new relationship and sharing the responsibility

A new baby will inevitably affect the relationship between a couple – not just temporarily, but permanently. Whether this is for the better depends very much on what each expects from the new situation, what each expects his or her role to be and the extent to which they both work at the very necessary adjusting and 'give and take' involved.

In the first few weeks, adapting to the new situation, routines and having the baby home may take more effort than anticipated. Few couples, of any age, can really anticipate just how great the strain caused by the changing relationship may be. There is no way of preparing for such events – they have to be lived through and experienced. Even though couples go through the pregnancy and birth itself together, often when the baby arrives there is a period during which this 'sharing' relationship is less harmonious. Sometimes parents become over-possessive about the child, which can build barriers between the two partners at a time when they need to strengthen their relationship. Even in this day and age fathers may still have an exaggerated pride in producing a son who is somehow 'theirs', or more special because of the association this has with passing on the family name. Mothers of baby daughters may exhibit similarly possessive behaviour. By laying claim to the child – 'my baby' or 'your baby' – they run the risk of undermining their own relationship and the new relationship with the child for whom they are both equally responsible. Feelings of jealousy,

rejection and simply not being needed may create stress for both partners.

But the very attachment of the mother to the baby through breast-feeding can make a husband or partner feel excluded, although this may be the last thing that the mother wants. In many ways the bonding process inevitably creates a strong tie between mother and child; that is what nature intended. But it also often means that, in the early months, the mother is the only one who can satisfy the baby's cravings – not just to be fed but also for the love and comfort which being held close to the mother's breast brings. It is not surprising, then, that men sometimes feel not just left out of this intensely close relationship, but also jealous of it.

Sometimes this strong tie which a mother who is breast-feeding feels causes some resentment on her part:

I got landed with a lot more because of the breast-feeding. I certainly had to cope with her at night every night. He took his share of bathing her, but the breast-feeding left me with a lot of it. She wouldn't ever take a bottle and I never got a morning or afternoon break from her to go shopping or anything like that. I suppose there is a slight touch of resentment there, but he has done his share in other ways. He does more now and is a considerable help in the evening.

It is quite easy to understand a situation in which a woman feels that, in providing love, care and physical support for her child, she is left with little energy to be the attractive loving wife at the end of the day. And it is quite easy to understand how her husband for his part simply sees the situation as one in which his attention and affection are rejected. But unless each can begin to tell the other how they feel, situations like this causes resentment which, if harboured and brooded over, can build into hardened attitudes – each seeing the other as unsympathetic and uncaring:

> He would come home in the evenings and I would be exhausted after being up in the night and up at six. I just wanted him to cook the supper and let me have an hour's rest. But he expected me to have it all ready and be full of life for the rest of the evening. He was so inconsiderate.

> She was totally engrossed in the baby and then when I got home in the evenings – I might just as well have not been there!

Inevitably, having a baby does bring a whole new dimension to a relationship which may provoke emotions that neither partner has felt before. It may be quite a jolt for a couple to discover that being a parent exposes them to all these new feelings. But they have to be able to respond to such feelings so that they can get on with the business of finding the best way to adjust to the new role of parent which adds to their relationship with their partner.

Allowing for all these new feelings and emotions and for the new situation to settle down into a bond that ties all three in a close, loving, family relationship requires time and patience. Perhaps,

also, willingness to talk more freely is the key to finding the balance:

> You think about the baby while you're pregnant, but you don't really think about how it's going to change your relationship. Tony and I have had a lot of arguments and we have disagreed about ways of coping with Peter. We didn't have a lot of time for each other – we were really tired for a long time and all of that was a big strain. But we have weathered it. We just weren't prepared for it. Maybe when you are older, though, you are that much more mature and you can talk through and work through the problems more easily.

Making love again

Many couples also look forward to the post-natal period and the pleasure of making love again, with the rosy prospect of the baby sleeping peacefully and contentedly in his cot: the reality may be far from that and it may take some time before sex is back on the agenda – despite post-natal check-ups and being given the 'all clear'. Needless to say, a number of factors are important here. If a woman has had tears and stitches she will want to feel comfortable and secure that these have healed. Some doctors advise that it is best to wait for the post-natal check-up. Others feel that how soon you make love again is for you to decide – when you are both ready for it. One study of 119 women showed that only 35 per cent had made love before the six weeks check. The study also showed that over half the women said they were less interested in sex three months after the birth than before pregnancy, and by a year after the birth 57 per cent of women were still not having sex as often as before.

For many couples, therefore, sex does present a problem in the weeks – or even months – after the birth. After the discomforts of later pregnancy and immediately after the birth, many men see no reason why making love should be postponed any longer. But a lot of women do not really want to have sexual intercourse for a long time after the baby is born, although they may want close physical contact. If a woman has had an episiotomy she may feel too uncomfortable. But even after this has completely healed many women do not enjoy making love for a number of reasons:

> I had the baby nursing every two or three hours, day and night. It seemed he was always latched onto my breast. After that I just didn't feel like anyone else making physical demands on me.

> I felt so emotionally upside down after the birth that I just couldn't cope with sex. I kept bursting into tears at the slightest thing and when we did make love I just got terribly upset.

Many women find that they do not feel very desirable as a new mother. Stretch marks, flabby tummy (at least initially), leaking breasts and clothes smelling of milk may make her feel the opposite of sexy, especially if she has always had time to take great care about her appearance. Some women have a deep seated feeling that mothers should not be sexy anyway. Others feel that their body belongs to the baby at this time and that anyone else is an intruder.

> I really didn't like sex in the early months – it really was a case of doing it for my husband's sake.

One recent study carried out on a small group of women has also suggested that breastfeeding has the effect of reducing a woman's interest in sex and that breastfeeding mothers are slower to resume intercourse after the birth, although the study does not offer any reasons why this should be so. It may be due to hormonal causes – breastfeeding women have a higher level of a hormone prolactin in their blood, which helps to suppress ovulation. However, it may also be that frequent waking for night feeds and resulting exhaustion may be the main cause – nursing mothers cannot hand-over to anyone else. Full tender breasts which leak as a result of pressure may also put a woman off making love:

> If I reached an orgasm my precious milk leaked out everywhere and I just felt nature didn't intend this really.

But a couple who want to resume their relationship can experiment with different positions which will avoid this problem and are comfortable for the woman.

Some women, especially breastfeeding mothers, find that the vagina does not lubricate so well for a time after the birth. If this is the case and you want to make love, it may help to use a lubricating jelly or cream.

Tiredness is also a factor reducing a couple's interest in sex, and this may affect the new father as much as the new mother. Waking for night feeds, walking up and down pacifying the baby – together with the emotional after-effects of birth and adjusting to the new routine, all take their toll. As one mother put it:

> When the baby settled and I fell into bed I used to nearly scream if Peter so much as touched me. I was so exhausted I couldn't afford to lose even five minutes sleep.

Some couples get round this problem by creating time for one another while the baby sleeps in the day, or when he is left with a relative or childminder.

> My mother used to take the baby out for a long walk so we had time for ourselves and we used to go to bed together – that was the only time we seemed to have.

Even if you are not ready for intercourse, it is important to find other ways of expressing your love and affection during the early weeks. Women who have had a lot of stitches or bruising may find they do not want to have full intercourse but other forms of sex are quite alright. Others are happier simply with caresses and cuddles. The feeling of closeness that a woman has with her new baby can make the husband feel left out, and it may be important that the woman recognizes this and is able to give the reassurance and sexual contact that he needs at this time, though it can be hard to balance the different needs men and women feel. If you wait till you do feel ready for sex, it will then probably come far more naturally than if you try to force things too soon.

When you do make love, it is important – even if you are fully breast-feeding – to use contraception, as it is easy to get pregnant soon after the birth of a baby. As well as this probably being the last thing you want, there are risks to both mother and baby if births are too closely spaced. (Those using a cap or IUD will have to wait until their post-natal check before they can be refitted.) Women are also usually advised to wait until the discharge after the birth (the lochia) has stopped – for some women this is not for six weeks or more.

If one partner wants to delay a return to their former sex life and the other does not, it can clearly be a cause of strain in a relationship. It is important to talk about your feelings honestly. Some people, perhaps especially men, see making love as a return to 'normal', to recover the kind of relationship that existed before the baby's birth. Of course, the relationship will have changed in some ways, and the time of adjustment may be quite difficult. By talking about your feelings and reaching some compromises, problems can be avoided:

> I never felt like making love, with a new baby and demanding toddler on my hands all day. But every so often I would take a deep breath and get on with it, and then I always thought, but this is really nice – why on earth don't we do it more often?

Sex, in fact, can act as a balm for frayed emotions and physical tiredness and set a seal on the new relationship between the couple and their baby. If you feel that your lack of interest in sex has gone on too long or it is causing problems in your relationship, or if you think it is a symptom of depression, then talk to your doctor about it.

Sharing the responsibility

From the practical point of view of getting things to run smoothly and the household 'ticking over', it does help if a clear pattern of roles and a fair division of responsibilities and duties is agreed. Attempts to share out the chores can end in confusion and conflict:

> At first we tried to involve ourselves in everything. This meant that we both got up for night feeds and both ended up completely exhausted. In the end we decided it was better if I did the night feeds since I had to get up anyway and he would take the baby off my hands first thing in the morning so I could have a lie in. Although in theory we wanted to share everything, we found in practice it just didn't work that way.

Some may find this time far more difficult to weather than others and they may not be able to resolve the 'sharing out' quite so easily:

> The biggest difficulty is with my husband. I think it's all right if you have sorted out your roles beforehand – he is Daddy and earns the money, you're Mummy and do the baby care. But we were both working and trying to do a bit of everything in a not very clearly defined way. So we ended up arguing all of the time. I would say, 'I have had a heavier day than you . . . so it's your turn to go to him and change his nappy.' And he would say, 'Yes, but I

spend more time at the office and I got up twice last night' . . . We were both so tired we were just trying to put as much as possible on to the other person, and the results were we were always trying to trade things off against the other. But you can't. Does two nappy changes equal one getting up in the night? . . . You just can't do it.

And it can be a time of real crisis for some couples:

> Of course, I wouldn't not have done it, and in many ways I feel better and happier than I have ever felt in my life. He is a wonderful joy to me. It's not motherhood itself that's so difficult, it's the combination of work and motherhood and marriage that doesn't seem so easy to get right.
> I'd like to live close by so that we can see one another, but not be on top of one another all the time. If we lived separately we could make our roles and responsibilities much clearer, I think – not this terrible muddle.

In practice, many couples find that the 'old fashioned' way of doing things still works best, although many men do take a much more active role in caring for the new baby – learning how to handle him, bath and feed him, change nappies and take their share of getting up at night: 'We don't share the domestic responsibilities because I am at home and I get on with it. I don't mind that. If I'm not doing anything else, it seems fair enough.'

While this may work well if the mother is at home full time, unless she feels confident that such arrangements are flexible, it may be a distinct drawback for a woman who is planning on returning to work:

> What worries me is if I were to take on a full-time job, it wouldn't change. I'd still be expected to do everything on top of that. Basically he just doesn't realize how much it entails. He thinks I should be able to slot it into a full-time job – partly because I did it before.

But for many couples the key is sharing out the chores and the responsibilities so that neither is tied and each feels satisfied with the arrangement:

> I usually get up at six or six-thirty. We work a rota system. I get up Monday to Friday and he gets up at the weekend. I get my tea in bed at the weekends so that gives me an hour or two longer lie. If you're up at eight instead of six it makes a big difference – it's sharing the routine. When he's away I have everything to do, but when he's here he baths her. After that is 'our time'. We usually just collapse sometimes with a drink and watch the 'telly'.

There are no hard-and-fast rules and no recipe to ensure that everyone lives 'happily ever after'. Traditional roles and responsibilities of both men and women have been well and truly questioned in recent years. Many women feel that being a wife and mother and having sole responsibility for the well-being of home and family is a hard lot and resent it. Likewise, many men have begun to question whether they don't lose out being the breadwinner. If there are lessons to be learned from these debates, it may simply be that both men and women need to be freed from the rigid constraints which have so sharply divided their roles in the past. Perhaps a few more men are staying home while the wife goes out to work. But these 'role reversals' seem to be little more than the old system in a new form. While they may be novel in themselves and demonstrate that men can provide the same sort of love and security traditionally provided by women, more men and more women are looking for more equal relationships. They want partnerships which do not deny one access to doing jobs other than in the home or the other a real share in the caring for and emotional development of children.

Whatever the rights and wrongs of these broad issues, in the final analysis it is the individual couple who have to work out a way of caring and providing for their family in a way that best suits them.

Yet beyond these individual issues of caring and coping, lies the fundamental joy of parenthood. To sum up in the words of one older mother.

> Nobody ever tells you how hard it is going to be – the pregnancy, the birth itself, the broken nights and hours of boredom and loneliness spent with your baby. Yet there is also tremendous joy in it, and nobody prepares you either for the kind of love relationship which blossoms with your baby and grows as your child becomes a person. So much is written about romantic love and very little about mothers' and fathers' love for their children – but I can think of nothing else so powerful,

or which leads you to do so many things you would otherwise hate, quite willingly to please them. Although I often moan – who doesn't – about how hard it is, I also know in my heart that having a baby is life's greatest experience and something I would never for a moment have missed.

Coming Late to Motherhood – Joan Michelson and Sue Gee (Thorsons 1984).

The Experience of Infertility – Naomi Pfeffer and Anne Woollett (Virago 1983)

It's Not Too Late For A Baby – For Women and Men over 35 – Sylvia P Reubin (Prentice-Hall 1980).

The New Birth Guide – Sheila Kitzinger (Penguin 1983).

Pregnancy and Childbirth – Sheila Kitzinger (Michael Joseph 1980, Reprinted Penguin 1986).

Pregnancy and Diet – Rachel Holme (Penguin 1985).

The Second Nine Months – The Sexual and Emotional Concerns of the New Mother. Judith M Gansburg and Arthur P Mostel (Thorsons, 1985).

Trying To Have a Baby – Overcoming infertility and child loss – Maggie Jones (Sheldon 1984).

When Pregnancy Fails. Coping with Miscarriage, Stillbirth and Infant Death – Susan Barg and Judith Laskel (Routledge Kegan Paul, 1982).

Working Through Your Pregnancy – Lee Rodwell (Thorsons, 1987).

Association for Improvements in the Maternity Services (AIMS)
163 Liverpool Road
London N1 0RF

A voluntary group which aims for improvements in the maternity services, giving advice about parents' rights, complaints procedures and choices in maternity care.

The Association for Post-Natal Illness
Institute of Obstetrics and Gynaecology
Queen Charlotte's Maternity Hospital
Goldhawk Road
London W6

Provides advice from mothers who have suffered from post-natal illness and have recovered, backed up by medical experts. A free leaflet on Post-natal depression is available if you send an s.a.e.

Association of Breastfeeding Mothers
131 Mayow Road
Sydenham
London SE26 4HZ
01 778 4769

Offers a 24-hour advice service to breastfeeding mothers and runs local support groups.

Community Health Councils (Local Health Councils in Scotland) Local CHC or LHC listed under local health authority in your phone book.

Will give advice on where and how to get the service you need and to help if you have a complaint.

Family Planning Information Service
27–35 Mortimer Street
London W1N 7RJ
01 636 7866

Information on methods of birth control as well as related matters such as infertility and sexual difficulties. Phone or write in for advice and information (s.a.e. appreciated).

Foresight
The Old Vicarage
Church Lane
Witley
Godalming
Surrey GU8 5PN
Tel: Wormley 4500

Provides information on how to prepare yourself for pregnancy, and offers genetic counselling.

Gingerbread
35 Wellington Street
London WC2E 7BN
01 240 0953

A self-help organization for one-parent families, with a network of local groups who offer support, information, advice and practical help.

La Leche League
BM 3424
London WC1 3XX
01 404 5011

Help and information to women who want to breastfeed their babies. Provides counsellors and also local groups hold informal talks on aspects of breastfeeding and parenthood. Send an s.a.e. for details of your nearest counsellor.

MAMA (Meet-a-Mum Association)
26a Cumnor Hill
Oxford
OX2 9HA

Moral support and practical help to women suffering from post-natal depression or feeling tired and isolated after having a child. To find your local group send an s.a.e. to above address.

The Maternity Alliance
59 Camden High Street
London NW1 7JL
01 388 6337

Provides information on all aspects of maternity care and rights. For free leaflets on benefits, maternity rights at work and health before pregnancy write sending an s.a.e.

National Caesarian Support Association
c/o Lynne Hallett
72 Perry Rise
London SE23 2QL
01 699 8339

Support and practical advice for women who have had, or may need, a Caesarian section.

National Childbirth Trust
9 Queensborough Terrace
Bayswater
London W2 3TB
01 221 3833

Runs antenatal classes giving information on methods of breathing and relaxation for childbirth and practical advice on breastfeeding. Local branches have postnatal support groups. Write or phone for more information and details of your nearest branch.

National Childminding Association
204–206 High Street
Bromley BR1 1PP
01 464 6164

An organization for childminders, child care workers, parents and anyone else with an interest in pre-school care, aiming to improve the status and conditions of childminders and the standard of care for children.

National Council for One Parent Families
255 Kentish Town Road
London NW5 2LX
01 267 1361

Free and confidential advice on matters relating to pregnancy, housing, social security, taxation, and maintenance. Write, phone or call in.

National Marriage Guidance Council
Herbert Gray College
Little Church Street
Rugby CV21 3AP
0788 73241

Confidential counselling for people with relationship problems of any kind. Local branch listed under Marriage Guidance in your phone book.

Pre-School Playgroups Association
Alford House
Aveline Street
London SE11 5DH
01 582 8871

A voluntary association of mother and toddler groups, playgroups and families of the under 5s who attend them. Provides help and support throughout England and Wales.

Twins Clubs Association
c/o Mrs D Hoeseason
Pooh Corner
54 Broad Lane
Hampton
Middlesex

A self-help organization to encourage and support parents of twins or more. Send an s.a.e. for details of membership and publications available.

Infertility

National Association for the Childless
318 Summer Lane,
Birmingham B19 3RL
021 359 4887

Provides advice, information and support to childless couples – both counselling for people with infertility problems and helping the childless to find a fulfilling lifestyle. Members can be referred to local groups. A newsletter and factsheet on childlessness are available on request.

British Pregnancy Advisory Service
Austy Manor,
Wooten Wawen,
Solihull,
West Midlands
05642 3225

BPAS provides counselling and infertility services for couples who find difficulty in obtaining the help they need through the National Health Service. They provide a full infertility investigation, AIH and AID, vasectomy and sterilization reversals, laparoscopy and tubal repair if necessary. A leaflet with more details and fees is available on request.

Child
'Farthings',
Pawlett,
Near Bridgwater,
Somerset
0278 683595

Provides information for those who are not able to conceive. A newsletter and factsheets are available. A 24-hour information service is available on the above number.

If you lose a baby

Compassionate Friends
5 Lower Clifton Hill
Clifton
Bristol BF8 1BT
0272 292778

Offers friendship and understanding to other bereaved parents.

The Foundation for the Study of Infant Deaths
(Cot Death Research and Support)
5th Floor
4 Grosvenor Place
London SW1 7HD
01 235 1721 or 245 9421

Gives support and information to parents whose baby dies suddenly.

The Miscarriage Association
Dolphin Cottage
4 Ashfield Terrace
Thorpe
Wakefield
West Yorkshire
0532 828946

Provides support, advice and information for women who have had or are having a miscarriage. For further information send an s.a.e.

Stillbirth and Neonatal Death Society (SANDS)
Argyle House
29–31 Euston Road
London NW1 2SD
01 833 2851/2

Provides information and support through a national network of support groups for bereaved parents. Phone or write for more details.

Support After Termination for Abnormality (SATFA)
22 Upper Woburn Place
London WC1H 0EP
01 388 1382

Provides information and support for women who have a pregnancy terminated because their baby has an abnormality. A newsletter is available on request.

Index

Abnormalities, screening for, 65-82
Abortion, 47, 49, 60, 80-2
Achondroplasia, 68
AID (Artificial Insemination by Donor), 16, 57-8
Alcohol, 27-8, 62
Alphafetoprotein Blood test, 72, 75-6, 78
Amniocentesis, 19, 35, 72, 75, 76-9, 81, 82
Amniotic fluid, 75, 76
Anencephaly, 68, 71, 75
Antenatal care, 37-42
Antenatal tests, 39-40
Antibiotics, 29
Antibodies, 52-3
Anti-nausea drugs, 29-30

Birth of baby, 83-104
Bonding, 95-6, 101-4
Breast feeding, 31, 105-9
—and bonding, 102
—and Caesarian section, 95, 106
—common problems, 108-9
—and Down's syndrome, 69
—and feelings, 130
—and premature baby, 98
—and sex, 132
Breathing techniques, 87

Caesarian section, 85-6, 89 92, 93-6, 102, 106
Calcium, 32, 34
Carbohydrates, 31-2
Cervical mucus, 44, 46-7, 52, 53
Cervical smear, 27, 39, 109
Cervix, 'incompetent', 63
Changes in birth practices, 38, 84, 101, 103-4
Child-minders, 121-2

Chorionic villi sampling, 72, 79
Chromosomes, 67-8
—abnormalities, 76, 79
Cleft palate and lip, 29, 68, 71-2
Conception, 44-5
Contraception
—after birth of baby, 133
—failed, 15-16
—and infertility, 49
—and post-natal check, 109
—stopping, 26-7
Contraceptive pill, 26, 29
Creches, 121
Cystic Fibrosis, 68

Depression
—antenatal, 41
—and infertility, 59
—post-natal, 110-11
Diaphragm 26, 27
Diet, 30-4, 71, 112-13
Digestive tract
—abnormalities, 72
Down's Syndrome, 35, 67, 68, 69-70, 76
Drugs, avoidance of, 27-30
Duchenne muscular dystrophy, 68, 81
Dysfunctional labour, 85

Emotional changes in
—pregnancy, 40-2
Endometrial biopsy, 53-4
Endometriosis, 50
Epidural anaesthesia, 87-9, 93, 95
Episiotomy, 86, 89, 90, 93, 132
Exercise in pregnancy, 35-7

Fallopian tube damage, 50
Fat, 32

Father, role of, 134-6
Fertile time, 45-7
Fertility drugs, 54-5
Fetoscopy, 72, 79
Fibre, 32
Fibroids, 50, 63
Foetal alcohol syndrome, 27-8
Foetal monitoring, 92
Forceps delivery, 86, 88, 92-3

Gas and air, 87
Genes, 67-8, 78
Genetic counselling, 34-5, 63
GIFT (gamete intra-fallopian transfer, 54, 55, 56

Haemophilia, 68, 81
Hormonal drugs, 29
Hormonal problems and
—deficiency, 49-50, 62-3
Huntingdon's Disease, 68
Hydrocephaly, 71
Hysterosalpingram, 54

Induction, 85, 91-2, 96
Infection, 27, 45, 50, 52
Infertility, 47-60
—causes of, 49-54
—tests, 53-4
—treatment for men, 56-8
—treatment for women, 54-6
Iron, 32, 34
Isolation, feelings of, 114
IUD, 26
IVF (in vitro fertilization), 54, 55, 56

Jaundice, 98
Jealousy, 115, 130

Labour
—beginning, 83-4
—difficult, 89-90
—pain relief in, 86-9
Laparoscopy, 54
Life-style, changes in, 24-5
Low birth-weight, 28, 32, 86, 96, 97, 98

Maternity leave and pay, 125-7
Minerals, 32
Miscarriage, 14, 17-18, 60-4
—causes of, 28, 61
—and genetic counselling, 35
—grief and loss, 61-2
—and older mother, 85, 86
—prevention of, 63-4
—and tests, 76, 77, 79
Mother-and-toddler group, 20, 114
Mumps, 45, 52

Nannies, 122-4
Neural tube defects, 68, 71, 75, 76, 78
Nurseries, 119, 121
Nutrients, essential, 33-4

Older children, 115-16
Older mother
—advantages of, 20-5
—feelings of, 13-14
—and isolation, 114
—and special risks in childbirth, 85-6
Organizations, 139-42
Ovulation, 44, 45, 46, 53, 54

Pain in labour, 83, 84, 86-9

—relief of, 86-9, 92
Painkillers, 28
Paternity leave, 126
Pelvic floor muscles, 36-7
Pethidine, 87
Phenylketonuria, 68
Planned pregnancy, 13-14
Post-coital test, 53, 54
Post-natal check, 109
Potassium, 32
Pre-eclampsia, 39-40, 85
Preconceptual care, 34-5
Premature baby, 42, 86, 93, 96-9
Preparation for pregnancy, 26-7
Protein, 31
Pudendal block, 89

Reactions to pregnancy, 17-18
Relationships after birth
—of baby, 130-6
Respiratory distress
    syndrome, 97
Rhythm method, 26

Screening for abnormalities, 65-82
Self-confidence, 20-1, 23, 114
Sex of baby, 72, 78-9
Sexual intercourse
—after birth of baby, 131-3
—and post-natal check, 109
—in pregnancy, 42
Sheath, 26, 27
Sicklecell Anaemia, 68
Smoking, 28, 49, 62
Sperm, 44, 46, 51-2
—production, 27, 52, 53, 56
Spermicides, 27

Spina Bifida, 68, 71, 75
Split ejaculate technique, 57
Stillbirth, 99-101
Stress and infertility, 59
Support, 106, 113-15
Surrogate motherhood, 56

Tay Sachs Disease, 68
Temperature chart, 46, 49, 53
Termination for abnormality, 80-2
Testerone rebound, 56
Testes and infertility, 52
Testicles, undescend, 52
Tiredness, 41, 42, 111-12
Trace elements, 32
Tranquillizers, 29
Tubal surgery, 55
Turner's Syndrome, 67
Twins, 40, 73, 75

Ultrasound scan, 35, 72-5
Unplanned pregnancy, 15-16

Varicocele, 52, 57
Ventouse, 93
Virility and infertility, 51
Vitamins, 32, 33, 71

Weight gain, 30-1, 39
Work
—and child care, 120-4
—freelance at home, 119
—part-time, 119
—returning to, 116-27
—as a strain, 42
—and weaning, 124-5

Zinc, 32, 34